**The Impact of Immigration on Children's Development**

# Contributions to Human Development

**Vol. 24**

Series Editor

**Larry Nucci** Berkeley, Calif.

# The Impact of Immigration on Children's Development

Volume Editor

**Cynthia Garcia Coll**  Providence, R.I.

8 figures and 16 tables, 2012

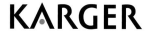

Basel · Freiburg · Paris · London · New York · New Delhi · Bangkok ·
Beijing · Tokyo · Kuala Lumpur · Singapore · Sydney

**Cynthia Garcia Coll**
Department of Education, Psychology and Pediatrics
Brown University
Providence, RI 02912, USA

Library of Congress Cataloging-in-Publication Data

The impact of immigration on children's development / volume editor, Cynthia Garcia-Coll.
    p. cm. -- (Contributions to human development ; v. 24)
  Includes bibliographical references and index.
  ISBN 978-3-8055-9798-2 (hbk. : alk. paper) -- ISBN 978-3-8055-9799-9 (electronic version)
  1. Immigrant children--Psychology. 2. Immigrant children--Social conditions. 3. Immigrants--Cultural assimilation. 4. Child psychology. 5. Child welfare.  I. García Coll, Cynthia T.
  JV6344.I47 2012
  304.8--dc23
                                                          2011036620

Bibliographic Indices. This publication is listed in bibliographic services, including Current Contents®.

Disclaimer. The statements, opinions and data contained in this publication are solely those of the individual authors and contributors and not of the publisher and the editor(s). The appearance of advertisements in the book is not a warranty, endorsement, or approval of the products or services advertised or of their effectiveness, quality or safety. The publisher and the editor(s) disclaim responsibility for any injury to persons or property resulting from any ideas, methods, instructions or products referred to in the content or advertisements.

Drug Dosage. The authors and the publisher have exerted every effort to ensure that drug selection and dosage set forth in this text are in accord with current recommendations and practice at the time of publication. However, in view of ongoing research, changes in government regulations, and the constant flow of information relating to drug therapy and drug reactions, the reader is urged to check the package insert for each drug for any change in indications and dosage and for added warnings and precautions. This is particularly important when the recommended agent is a new and/or infrequently employed drug.

All rights reserved. No part of this publication may be translated into other languages, reproduced or utilized in any form or by any means electronic or mechanical, including photocopying, recording, microcopying, or by any information storage and retrieval system, without permission in writing from the publisher.

© Copyright 2012 by S. Karger AG, P.O. Box, CH–4009 Basel (Switzerland)
www.karger.com
Printed in Switzerland on acid-free and non-aging paper (ISO 9706) by Reinhardt Druck, Basel
ISSN 0301-4193
ISBN 978-3-8055-9798-2
e-ISBN 978-3-8055-9799-9

# Contents

**VII Introduction: The Global, the Local – Children and Immigration around the World**
Garcia Coll, C. (Providence, R.I./Puerto Rico)

**1 Quiet in the Eye of the Beholder: Teacher Perceptions of Asian Immigrant Children**
Yamamoto, Y.; Li, J. (Providence, R.I.)

**17 The Impact of Social Contexts in Schools: Adolescents Who Are New to Canada and Their Sense of Belonging**
Gagné, M.H.; Shapka, J.D.; Law, D.M. (Vancouver, B.C.)

**35 Are Immigrant Children in Italy Better Adjusted than Mainstream Italian Children?**
Dimitrova, R.; Chasiotis, A. (Tilburg)

**49 Ethnic Identity, Acculturation Orientations, and Psychological Well-Being among Adolescents of Immigrant Background in Kenya**
Abubakar, A. (Tilburg/Utrecht); van de Vijver, F.J.R. (Tilburg/Potchefstroom); Mazrui, L.; Arasa, J.; Murugami, M. (Nairobi)

**64 Immigrant Youth Adaptation in Context: The Role of Society of Settlement**
Sam, D.L. (Bergen); Horenczyk, G. (Jerusalem)

**77 Examining Spiritual Capital and Acculturation across Ecological Systems: Developmental Implications for Children and Adolescents in Diverse Immigrant Families**
Oh, S.S.; Yoshikawa, H. (Cambridge, Mass.)

**99 Immigrant Youth and Discrimination**
Vedder, P.; van Geel, M. (Leiden)

**122 Immigrant Family Separations: The Experience of Separated, Unaccompanied, and Reunited Youth and Families**
Suárez-Orozco, C.; Hernández, M.G. (New York, N.Y.)

**149 Author Index**
**150 Subject Index**

# Introduction: The Global, the Local – Children and Immigration around the World

Cynthia Garcia Coll

Brown University, Providence, RI, USA, and University of Puerto Rico, San Juan, Puerto Rico

Migration and immigration have been part of human history since ancient times. Individuals, families and groups migrate for a variety of reasons, from escaping war, persecution and famine to enhancement of life prospects. It is a complex phenomenon that depends very much on the individual migrant as well as the contexts of the sending and receiving communities. The growth of migrant populations in recent history has led receiving countries to enact policies ranging from dedicated resources to support immigrants' adaptation to punitive ones for their arrival.

Currently, immigration is a worldwide phenomenon. Through technological connections, the world economies and cultures are intertwined at a larger and more immediate scale than ever before. This has led to a variety of migration patterns that are characterized as transnational, seasonal, revolving door or lead to permanent settlements. Many countries are affected by either being a source or recipients of migrants or both. At first glance, similarities across countries arise in the factors that affect the immigration process: the economy and political stability of the countries of origin as a major pushing factor; attitudes toward immigrants and perceived opportunities for education and social mobility as actual employment opportunities as pull factors.

The purpose of this book is to give a glance of how this phenomenon impinges on children's development. Children are either brought along and are part of the migration process itself or are born into the new countries to immigrant families. Regardless of their birth site, these children all have in common the experience of having a family who originated in another country and are now living in another. Potential clashes in patterns of behaviors, beliefs and morality, of how to sustain a family, of childrearing practices and goals are all particular issues that all immigrant parents face in the new lands. Children on the other hand have to learn how to negotiate multiple worlds, how to create continuities when there are none, how to become competent in the outside world with little guidance from their parents and other family members. They might be faced with contradictory messages, even some rather incompatible ones and with racism and discrimination based on their religion, color of their skin or even their accent or culturally defined mannerisms. In sum, issues of adaptation to new contexts are universal to the experience of growing up in an immigrant family.

Yet besides those very general glances at the global aspects of migration, each immigrant story presents a slice of reality quite different from another. To talk about the immigrant experience in general is to gloss over a lot of particularities that are significant sources of variance in the adaptation of children from immigrant backgrounds. The continuities and discontinuities between the country of origin and the recipient in culture, language, life skills, employment, language, sex roles, religion, racial profile, etc. become major sources of variability for migrants and for their adaptations over time. So do the policies toward incorporation from the receiving country as well as the public perception of immigrants as assets or burdens or both to the society at large. These policies and other historical factors can contribute to segregation and lack of opportunities and access to critical educational, health and employment opportunities. Who migrates, who stays behind and how much contact is maintained with the country of origin varies widely by the context of migration and the relationship between the two countries and the particular migrant group's history of settlement. Migrants are also many times thought of as a self-selected group that might differ from those who stay behind in important ways. Finally, immigrants also differ in their level of education, social class, trauma, race, age and gender, and many other demographic characteristics that contribute to further variation. Thus not only contextual, cultural, economic, and political forces impinge on the immigrant experience but personality and individual agency is very much part of the impetus for migrating and subsequent adaptation. These sources of variation are important to consider when we examine the impact of migration on children's development.

As the immigrant populations have increased in most developed countries, the most dominant world view is of immigrant populations struggling all over the world and of failing to be successful in adapting to the new cultures and economies. The media has been avid to depict the unrest of young immigrants and their lack of success in conventional terms in the new countries. A rise of anti-immigrant popular sentiments and policies have swept the developed world in response to an immigrant tide that is seeing as eroding national values and quality of life. These views are partly true and reflect the experiences of some immigrant groups and individuals. But the story is more complicated than that.

Recent research including the one included in this book, documents outcomes as varied as the intersections of the many reception and sending variables as well as individual factors mentioned before. We see immigrant children for example finishing at the top of their class in disproportionate numbers in spite of many obstacles. At the same time, we see some included in the unacceptable high numbers of school dropouts. The patterns of adaptation observed range from excelling to complete failure and everything in between. Sociologist have created concepts like segmented assimilation to depict different ways of adaptation that include the adoption of values and behavior patterns that are associated with living in poverty and derailing many immigrant parents' dreams as well as successful ones. The phenomena of the immigrant paradox, the fact that successive generations or more advanced acculturation within immigrant populations is associated with more negative outcomes has also received attention in the areas of health, education and risky behaviors. The documentation of outcomes is now leading to investigations of why we see the sometimes even extremes of adaptations amongst immigrant groups and their children. In sum, the newspaper headlines miss the nuances of individuals and immigrant groups and the extent of variability observed in developmental outcomes.

One of the main variables that impinge on these outcomes is age at migration; developmental processes interact with migration and adaptation in very profound ways. For example, the new host country might have a very different language than the sending one. Learning the new language will be a different task depending on the age of the migrant: it is much easier the younger the person, but at what cost? Can bilingualism and biculturalism, outcomes that are seen as positive in some countries (i.e. the United States of America) be maintained with the exposure to the host countries' culture very early on?

Much of the literature on migration have documented adaptation processes in adults; much less is known about children and adolescents, and most books with younger populations tend to be in one immigrant group or in one country. This book is intended to open the field to include various countries, both experienced and inexperienced with migration. Our purpose is to bring together perspectives from various countries and immigrant groups into the study of adaptations that children from immigrant backgrounds have to do. The presentation of a variety of perspectives is intended to identify both commonalities and differences across contexts: the global and the local. There are common threads across groups and contexts, and then they are unique assets and demands. For example, all children have to adapt to the new culture; only a percentage of them have to deal with being separated from parents at some point in their journey. What we learn immediately when we take the universe of observations is the difficulty of making generalizations across contexts and immigrant groups. A balanced accurate view of these adaptations requires the identification of both universal (global) and community (local)-defined pathways and the strengths and weaknesses of the immigrant him-/herself in the context of reception. These are not individual stories, but neither are they common to all individuals in one group or across groups or nations.

The book also intends to highlight some of the most basic contextual processes that impinge on the development of children and adolescents from immigrant backgrounds. Schools, religion, parental separation, discrimination are all part of the context of immigration and reception, important variables to study as we try to understand the variability observed in developmental outcomes. Understanding contextual factors as well as individual ones is a must in this area. We hope that this book stimulates going beyond documenting developmental outcomes to a systematic analysis of the factors that explain such findings.

As native populations in developed countries slow down their fertility, these countries have looked at immigrant populations as sources of work and future growth. Unfortunately, mutual adaptations have been harder than expected by both sides. Children and adolescent are usually caught in the middle of these battles where adults take decisions that impinge on their lives with very little or no consultation or consideration of the youth's needs. Policies are enacted by adults and for adults in many respects. But we have the power to change this. We hope that this book will contribute to an awareness of the many unique needs of children from immigrant backgrounds, inclusive not only of their struggles but also of their strengths.

# Quiet in the Eye of the Beholder: Teacher Perceptions of Asian Immigrant Children

Yoko Yamamoto · Jin Li

Department of Education, Brown University, Providence, R.I., USA

## Abstract

Cultural norms and practices that are brought by immigrant families may engender advantages or disadvantages to immigrant children's development and school experiences. Extensive research shows that Asian immigrant children achieve well in general owing to the ways Asian immigrant families socialize their children. However, research has also found Asian children to be shy, quiet or silent in class and school. While quietness can be viewed as a positive attitude which reflects students' attentive listening and sensitivity to others in East Asia, it may be perceived negatively in Western schools, where self-expression is valued. The present study examined teachers' perceptions about Chinese immigrant children's verbal expressions compared to European Americans' (EA) at an early stage. We also examined how teachers' assessment of children's verbal expression is related to the child's school adjustment, peer relations, learning engagement, and academic performance in two distinctive school contexts: Asian-dominant and EA-dominant preschools. Data included achievement tests with 166 4-year-olds (59 low-socioeconomic status Chinese, 49 middle-class Chinese, and 58 middle-class EA) and surveys from their teachers. Results demonstrated that teachers viewed Chinese immigrant children to be significantly quieter and less expressive than EA children. In Asian-dominant preschools, quietness was associated with better school adjustment and learning engagement. In EA-dominant preschools, Chinese immigrant children's quietness was associated with negative peer relations and learning engagement. Self-expressions or quietness was not correlated with children's academic performance after controlling for socioeconomic status. We present hypotheses and pathways to interpret and explain our findings.

Copyright © 2012 S. Karger AG, Basel

Kai's mother attended a parent-teacher conference and was shocked by the preschool teacher's comments. The European American teacher said that Kai, who had been at the preschool for 6 months, is quiet and reserved. She reported that he usually watches other children play and does not express what he wants. The teacher advised his mother to encourage Kai to express his needs and ideas verbally at home. Kai's mother wondered why the teacher would not facilitate Kai and other children to play together or ask what he wanted to make his school life smooth, as teachers in East Asia would do. The mother was also surprised at the negative image of quietness presented to her. In her country of origin, young children's shyness and quietness are considered to be natural or even positive since these characteristics indicate the child's sensitivity to others.

Hearing a European American (EA) teacher make negative comments about her child's quietness is not unique to Kai's mother but rather relatively common among Asian immigrant parents. In fact, Asian children's quietness, along with the cultural origin and psychological effects of quietness, has been of interest to researchers for several decades. Although commonly experienced and studied as a personality flaw, quietness may be more complex than previously understood. Once reconceptualized, the quietness of Asian immigrant children may surprise us by its contextual oscillation from school to school or from home to school. Whether quietness is negative or positive may indeed reside in the eyes of the beholders of different cultural backgrounds.

In this chapter, we review research literature on cultural norms and attitudes toward quietness and self-expression/assertiveness in East Asia and the West. We focus on children's school outcomes as a function of these cultural differences. Next, we propose a new conceptual framework with which to reexamine Asian immigrant children's quietness: shifting the perspective of quietness as a child's fixed personality flaw to the dynamic functioning of his or her school and social contexts. Then, we report our empirical support for such a framework shift. Based on the patterns found, we further highlight a set of mediators through which quietness or self-expression may promote or inhibit children's school experiences and their socioemotional development in different school contexts. Finally, we conclude by calling for more research into contextual dynamics when examining school experiences and the development of Asian immigrant children.[1]

## Cultural Norms and Children's School Experiences

Cultural norms and practices of immigrant families may foster advantages or disadvantages for immigrant children's development. Whether a given cultural norm or practice presents an advantage or disadvantage is related to the immigrant context in which the norms and practices of home culture and host culture interact [García, Coll & Marks, 2009].

Asians were the fastest growing racial group in the US between 2000 and 2010 [US Census Bureau, 2011]. In 2010, Asian Americans numbered approximately 14.7 million [US Census Bureau, 2011]. Between 1965 and 2002, about 8.3 million Asian immigrants were admitted to permanent residency, which consisted of 34% of all immigrants [US Census Bureau, 2007]. Extensive research has demonstrated that, generally, children of Asian immigrant parents are high academic achievers [Kao, 1995; Suárez-Orozco, Suárez-Orozco & Todorova, 2008; Zhou & Kim, 2006]. Asian Americans as well as Asian immigrants have acquired the reputation of being 'a model minority' in various Western countries due to their high academic performance and positive attitudes toward education [Archer & Francis, 2005; Li & Wang, 2008; Ng, Lee & Pak, 2007]. Such high academic performance has been explained within the context of Asian immigrant families socializing their children and the resources they deploy to contribute to their children's schooling. As a rule, Asian immigrant parents highly value education, hold high expectations for their children's education, and provide academic support for their children's educational progress [Hao & Bornstead-Bruns, 1998; Sy & Schulenberg, 2005; also see Yamamoto & Holloway, 2010].

However, highlighting these positive practices and norms conceals difficulties and challenges experienced by Asian immigrant children in Western schools. First, not all Asian children do well in school. Due to the model minority stereotype, Asian immigrant children who suffer academic difficulties are likely to be neglected and to receive limited support and attention [see Li & Wang, 2008]. Second, ample evidence has demonstrated that the school experience of Asian immigrant children is filled with obstacles, including a high rate of peer

---

[1] We use the term 'Asian immigrant children' to indicate both Asian immigrant children who themselves experienced migration and children in Asian immigrant families who were born in the host country even though we recognize the difference between them. The majority of participants in our research consisted of children in chinese immigrant families who were born in the US, but our participants also included Chinese children who came to the US before age 4.

harassment and discrimination, that are linked to social alienation and depression [Kao, 1999; Qin, Way & Mukherjee, 2008]. As Bankston and Zhou [2002] pointed out, doing well in school is different from being well in school. Third, researchers have discovered that Asian immigrant children are quiet or silent in Western classrooms and schools [Archer & Francis, 2005; Liu, 2002]. In fact, stereotypes of Asian students by Western teachers and students include 'silent', 'quiet', 'passive', 'non-assertive', and 'poor communicators' [Kim, 2002; Kim & Yeh, 2002; Lei, 2003; Liu, 2002; Mathews, 2000]. As illustrated by Kai's mother's anecdote, and as we describe in the next section, cultural expectations for verbal expression in East Asia and the West are distinct. Thus, learning two distinct sets of norms related to verbal expression is likely to become a source of acculturative stress or struggle for Asian immigrant children as they transition from home to school. While psychological studies have documented the role of quietness in children's socioemotional development within East Asian and Western cultural contexts, little is known about how quietness or self-expression affects school experiences and learning processes among Asian immigrant children, especially during the preschool and early school years. It is particularly important to understand how Western teachers perceive verbal expression among Asian immigrant children versus native children and how such views affect young children's school experiences and academic processes. In this chapter, we explore two distinct forms of communication styles, quietness versus self-expression, to examine school experiences and academic processes among Asian immigrant children in the US.

## Quietness versus Self-Expression in East Asia and the West

The meanings of quietness, self-expression, and related behavior differ significantly from culture to culture. Quietness as well as self-expression can become a positive or negative communication style depending on cultural contexts [Tannen & Saville-Troike, 1985]. In East Asia, quietness and shyness are considered to be virtues because such characteristics demonstrate caution, modesty, and courtesy, indicating a valued sensitivity to social environments [Azuma, 1986; Chen, Chen, Li & Wang, 2009; Li, in press]. In cultures that emphasize non-confrontational interpersonal relations, intuitive communication is critical; these cultures value ambiguity in social and public relationships and often encourage people to restrain verbal expression [Lebra, 1976; Liu, in press]. Asserting one's needs tends to be perceived as selfish or immature since it indicates a lack of sympathy, modesty, and ability to express one's thoughts with sensitivity to others. Children are expected to learn the importance of the context of expression, including whether they should keep quiet or talk in specific situations [Ishii & Bruneau, 1994; Lebra, 1987]. This learning about context becomes a critical skill at school in East Asia. Being quiet, especially self-imposed silence, is considered positive in relation to teachers because it demonstrates respect for the teacher, who is generally perceived to be an authority [Holloway & Yamamoto, 2003; Liu, 2002].

When a student disagrees with the teacher and challenges the teacher in class, the student's behavior is likely to be perceived by his or her peers as well as the teacher as seeking attention for the self or showing off. Those behaviors may be considered inappropriate and may damage the group atmosphere or others' feelings. Children in East Asia learn to be cautious and not to express disagreement or challenging ideas directly. However, this cultural norm does not mean that East Asian children can never express their disagreement or opinion. They simply express these feelings in a different style, such as talking to the teacher one-on-one, talking to peers in group work, or writing in journals [Inagaki, Hatano & Morita, 1998; Li & Sklar, 2010].

These cultural values of quietness and restraint of self-assertion are reflected in parenting styles and children's socialization processes in East Asia. For example, Japanese mothers vocalize less to their infants than EA mothers [Caudill & Weinstein, 1969]. Moreover, toddlers' inhibited behavior is positively associated with encouragement to achieve among Chinese mothers, whereas such associations are negative among European Canadian mothers [Chen et al., 1998]. Furthermore, East Asian parents tend to encourage children to improve their skills in reading and interpreting others' feelings and desires without directly asking questions. Examinations of mother-child conversations document that Japanese mothers request fewer descriptions and elaborations in their children's speech compared to American mothers [Minami, 1994; Minami & McCabe, 1995; Murase, Dale, Ogura, Yamashita & Mahieu, 2005]. Finally, East Asian mother-child communication stresses the child's ability to listen. Accordingly, children are socialized to listen attentively before they speak. Listening attentively also shows respect for the social context. When children speak, they need to speak appropriately within the context (e.g. when adults ask them a question or when they discern that their speaking is expected). Speaking out of context or disrespectfully not only reflects poorly on the child him-/herself, but also on the child's family [Li, in press; Miller, Fung, Lin, Chen & Boldt, in press]. Although East Asian parents also encourage their children to express their feelings and thoughts, especially to their mothers [Holloway, 2010], Asian children are likely to internalize the values associated with quietness and believe that quietness is an appropriate or desired social practice in certain contexts based on their day-to-day interactions with their parents.

In contrast, expressing one's thoughts and feelings explicitly and asserting one's desires and needs are expected, valued, or even necessary in Western societies. Self-expression and assertiveness is not only regarded as a personal intellectual quality, but also as a political right and an indication of leadership skill and charisma [Li, in press]. Eloquence and self-assertion has a positive connotation in the US and Europe, often viewed as opposite from being quiet, and 'the more speaking, the better – at home, at school, and in business' [Ishii & Bruneau, 1994, p. 250]. Verbal communication is a tool for interpersonal understanding in a society where people view individuals as independent and different [Markus & Kitayama, 1991]. Silence or quietness is often viewed negatively, especially in social relationships and public settings such as school [Ishii & Bruneau, 1994; Tannen & Saville-Troike, 1985].

Such a cultural emphasis guides Western parents to focus on nurturing self-assertion in children's socialization processes. Middle-class adults expect children to utter their messages verbally and elaborate them rather than restraining or simplifying them. Children have the right to express their individuality and are asked by adults their wishes and desires. An ethnographic study conducted by Lareau [2003] illustrated processes through which middle-class American children learn to express their desires and debate with adults through the use of reason, even at a young age. Through interactions with parents in daily life, middle-class American children learn that they have 'a right to weigh in with an opinion, to make special requests, to pass judgment on others, and to offer advice to adults' (p. 133). Lareau argued that such verbal skills are a form of 'cultural capital' that accrues benefits when children attend school because American society 'places a premium on assertive, individualized actions executed by persons who command skills in reasoning and negotiation' (p. 133).

*Asian Quietness Meets Western Self-Expression in School Contexts*
What happens then when Asian children's quietness meets Western self-expression in school? Although abundant cross-cultural studies have demonstrated distinct verbal and communication styles in East Asia and the West, we know very little about how Asian immigrant children fare in Western schools when displaying their quiet characteristic. This question relates to the

acculturative process that both parents and children undergo and the associated impact on Asian immigrant children's learning and school adjustment. Immigrant parents, especially middle-class parents, are likely to be exposed to American values regarding verbal skills through interaction and communication with American coworkers, neighbors, or family members. Yet, we do not know whether parents' exposure to American values and communication modes influences their parenting styles to make them encourage their children to be less quiet and more elaborative and assertive in their speech. As Cheah and Leung [2011] pointed out, some cultural practices change in accordance with acculturation processes, but others are resistant to change. In order for immigrant parents to change their culturally based parenting practice, the parents have to perceive the new practice shared in a host country as positive and beneficial to their children and the family members.

Possessing a certain cultural norm is not the sole determinant of positive or negative school experiences of immigrant children. Actors in schools, such as teachers and peers in the host country, evaluate the cultural norms brought by the immigrant families and provide positive or negative feedback to the children that influences their school experiences. Children's quietness is likely to be interpreted differently depending on the sensitivity of teachers and other students to understanding the act of silence. Furthermore, in some context quietness is welcomed, but in others it is considered to be negative.

In East Asian classrooms, quietness reflects students' attentive listening, active thinking, and ability to solve problems independently [Takeishi, 2008]. Asking questions in the middle of class is considered to be inappropriate and disturbing. However, students are expected to ask questions after class or express their responses clearly when teachers initiate questions [Liu, 2002]. Asian teachers also view quiet children as hard workers since they believe that action originates when people do not talk [Davies & Ikeno, 2002]. Thus, Asian teachers and students do not necessarily view the expression of ideas or participation in discussions as a key academic competence or active engagement in learning [Liu, 2002].

Children of Asian immigrant families are likely to face a difficult adjustment at the time of transition from home to school in Western countries because school cultures represent Western norms. Western teachers may view silent behavior among Asian immigrant students as a lack of interests or knowledge [Liu, 2002; Remedios, Clarke & Hawthorne, 2008]. In American schools, teachers view verbal communication skills as representative of an active mind, engaged learning, and academic competence. Western teachers expect students to demonstrate their ideas and speak up in classrooms [McCroskey & Daly, 1976]. Quietness can be interpreted to mean a lack of understanding, independent thinking, and low intelligence [Liu, 2002; McCroskey, 1980]. While little empirical evidence has demonstrated the consequences of being quiet in school among Asian immigrant children, cross-cultural studies have shown that quiet children receive more negative emotional and social sanctions in Western schools [Chen et al., 2009; Hart et al., 2000]. In China, shy or inhibited behavior is not associated with negative social and emotional outcomes such as depression in school-aged children, but this association is documented among Western children [Chen, Rubin & Li, 1995]. An early study by Rubin and Mills [1988] reported that children's passiveness at the second grade is associated with peer rejection, internalized difficulties, negative social perceptions, and later depression and loneliness in Canada. These studies suggest that Western school contexts may inhibit the healthy development of quiet and shy children.

*The Present Study*
We examined these issues in the preschool period, the first 'ecological transition' or transition from home to school [Bronfenbrenner, 1979]. While not all children attend preschool, more than two

thirds of children in the US do [Barnett, Epstein, Friedman, Sansanelli & Hustedt, 2009]. For a large number of children of immigrants, preschool is the first environment in which they are exposed to the mainstream culture. Therefore, preschool is one of the most critical periods in understanding the developmental and acculturation processes of immigrant children [Marks, Patton & García Coll, 2010]. Yet, most studies on Asian immigrant children have focused on adolescence, and little attention has been paid to this early period.

Our assumption is that school and academic experiences among immigrant children are more complex than those of native-born children because immigrant children are likely to receive conflicting messages regarding verbal expression at home and school. However, variations within the Asian immigrant group also may exist. Asian immigrant children who live in ethnic enclaves and attend schools where the majority of teachers and peers are Asians are likely to have different experiences from those attending schools in which most of the actors are non-Asians. Thus, in addition to examining Chinese immigrant (CI) children and native-born EA children, we investigated two different school contexts for CI children, Asian-dominant and EA-dominant preschools, to understand how quiet and assertive children have different school experiences depending on the ethnic composition of the school. The goal of this study was to provide general perceptions of teachers about CI children's communication styles and to report patterns associated with CI children's quietness and verbal expression. Therefore, we focused on presenting descriptive findings rather than testing specific hypotheses.

**Teacher Perceptions and Patterns: Quietness of Chinese Immigrant Children**

*Method and Procedure*
Data for this study came from an ongoing longitudinal study which examined the development of learning beliefs among CI and EA children. We recruited the children and families from daycare centers, preschools, and organizations in urban and suburban areas of the states of Massachusetts and Rhode Island, both in the North Eastern coast of the United States. The parents received recruitment packets and signed consent forms for participation. For the current study, we examined 166 4-year-olds (59 CI of low socioeconomic status (SES), 49 middle-class CI, and 58 middle-class EA). The majority of parents of CI children migrated from China, but some came from Hong Kong or Taiwan. All but 9 CI children were born in the US. CI mothers in this study had lived in the US for 9.7 years on average (SD = 5.7), and there was no significant difference in US residency among CI mothers between the low-SES and middle-class groups or between Asian-dominant or EA-dominant preschools.

Participants included 82 boys and 84 girls. There was no significant difference in gender ratio across low-SES CI, middle-class CI, and EA groups. We defined parents' SES using Hollingshead index scores [Hollingshead, 1975]. Low-SES parents had a score below 40, were engaged in a low-wage job, and did not have a college education. Middle-class parents had a score of 40 or above, were typically engaged in white-collar or professional work, and had at least an undergraduate college education. Fifty-two of the CI children attended a preschool in which more than 50% of the teachers were EA (hereafter EA-dominant preschool). Most of these schools were located in suburbs. Fifty-six CI children attended a preschool in which more than 50% of the teachers were Asians, mostly Chinese, such as preschools and family care facilities owned by Asian people and centers and Head Start located in Chinatown (hereafter Asian-dominant preschool). The two types of preschools reflected social class differences. Seventy-five percent of CI children who attended EA-dominant preschools had middle-class backgrounds compared to 18% of CI children who attended Asian-dominant preschools.[2] All EA children attended EA-dominant preschools.

We conducted interviews with children and their parents and collected evaluations from children's classroom teachers. Teachers rated each child's quietness, self-expression/assertiveness (hereafter self-expression).[3] Teachers also assessed children's school adjustment by evaluating their emotional and behavioral difficulties at school. Furthermore, teachers rated peer relations and learning engagement.[4] We administered the Woodcock-Johnson achievement test to assess children's academic performance in math and reading.[5] To evaluate their English proficiency, we conducted the Pre-LAS English test [Duncan & De Avila, 1998] with CI children.[6] We also interviewed children's parents and acquired demographic information such as parent education, occupation, and mothers' length of US residency (for CI only).

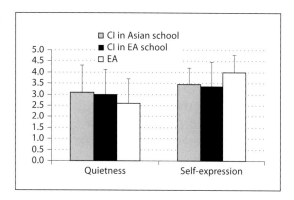

**Fig. 1.** Teachers' ratings for quietness and self-expression for CI children in Asian-dominant preschools and EA-dominant preschools and EA children.

## Summary of Findings

*Do Teachers View CI Children as Quieter and Less Expressive?*
Preschool teachers, regardless of their ethnic backgrounds, rated CI children as being significantly less expressive/assertive, t(164) = 4.13, p < 0.001, and quieter, t(160) = –2.33, p = 0.02, than EA children, even at age 4 (fig. 1). We found the same pattern when we compared only middle-class CI children to EA children. There was no significant difference in teacher perception of CI children's quietness and self-expression between Asian-dominant and EA-dominant preschools or between middle-class and low-SES groups. CI girls were perceived to be quieter than CI boys in Asian-dominant preschools, t(52) = –2.55, p = 0.014, but no gender difference was found for CI and EA children attending EA-dominant preschools.

These findings demonstrate that according to teacher ratings, CI children appear to be or are perceived to be quieter and less expressive than EA children regardless of the type of preschool attended or children's SES backgrounds.

*Are Acculturation and English Proficiency Associated with Children's Quietness or Self-Expression?*
One way to measure parents' acculturation level is by their length of US residency even though this measurement is not a true reflection of their acculturation since some immigrant parents may not interact or communicate with native people despite a lengthy US residence [Alegria, 2009]. Length of

---

[2] We controlled for SES, either middle class or low-SES, in all subsequent analyses.
[3] To assess children's quietness, we asked teachers to rate if the child is quiet using a 5-point scale (1, rarely applies, to 5, always applies). Self-expression was a mean score of teacher ratings for children's verbal assertiveness such as expression of feelings and verbal assertion of needs and desires based on a 5-point scale (4 items).
[4] Peer relations was a mean score of 5 items assessing children's relationships with other students. Learning engagement was a mean score of 29 items assessing children's attitudes and behaviors toward learning (see appendix).
[5] We used a mean score of standardized scores for math and reading.
[6] Pre-LAS is a test designed to measure young children's abilities of listening and speaking in English. An interviewer administered Pre-LAS for an individual child and identified a proficiency level ranging from 1 to 5 based on the total score.

mothers' residence in the US was not associated with children's quietness or self-expression among CI children, even when we looked at the correlation within each type of preschool.[7] We also examined how CI children's English proficiency was associated with their verbal expression. We found that English proficiency was not associated with CI children's expression/assertion or quietness. However, the relationship between CI children's English proficiency and self-expression appeared to vary depending on the type of school. English proficiency was positively correlated with CI children's self-expression, $r(51) = 0.33$, $p = 0.018$ (2-tailed), but not with quietness, even after controlling for SES, in EA-dominant preschools. There were no correlations among English proficiency, quietness, and self-expression in Asian-dominant preschools. Thus, CI children's quietness or expressiveness is not likely to be associated with their mother's length of US residence. However, the better CI children's English is, more expressive they become in EA-dominant preschools. Since language proficiency is used very frequently as a measure of the individual's level of acculturation, it may capture this process better than mother's length of US residence.

*Verbal Expressions and Child Outcomes across the Three Groups*
There was no significant difference in any of the child outcome variables between CI children attending an EA-dominant preschool and EA children. We also found no significant difference in child outcome variables between CI children in Asian-dominant preschools and CI children in EA-dominant preschools after controlling SES. Next, we examined how quietness and self-expression were associated with child outcome variables by conducting partial correlation analysis tests with SES as a control within each group: CI in Asian-dominant preschools, CI in EA-dominant preschools, and EA (table 1). Since there was no gender difference in any outcome variables for all groups, we did not further examine this issue.

*CI Children in Asian-Dominant Preschools.* In Asian-dominant preschools, quietness was positively associated with teachers' ratings regarding school adjustment and learning engagement. The significant correlation between quietness and academic performance disappeared after controlling SES. Self-expression was correlated with positive peer relations and higher learning engagement (see table 1).

*CI Children in EA-Dominant Preschools.* In EA-dominant preschools, self-expression was positively correlated with school adjustment, peer relations, and learning engagement. Quietness was negatively correlated with peer relations and learning engagement in this type of preschool.

*EA Children.* We found similar patterns between EA children and CI children attending EA-dominant preschools. However, the quietness was not significantly correlated with peer relations and learning engagement. Self-expression was positively correlated with school adjustment, peer relations, and learning engagement. We also found a negative correlation between quietness and self-expression.

## Interpretations and Suggested Mediators

*Quiet and Less Expressive Chinese Immigrant Children*
Our results demonstrated that CI children are perceived to be quieter and less expressive than EA children by their teachers, regardless of teacher ethnic background. Due to the stereotype of Asian children as quiet, it is possible that many teachers perceive CI children to be quieter than others. However, we speculate that CI children might actually be quieter and less expressive/assertive at school than EA children because socialization processes among CI families do not emphasize the development of self-expression and

---

[7] We ran the Pearson correlation analyses to examine these associations.

**Table 1.** Summary of partial correlations among quietness, self-expression, peer relations, school adjustment, learning engagement, and academic performance among CI children in Asian-dominant and EA-dominant preschools and EA children

| CI in Asian-dominant schools | 1 | 2 | 3 | 4 | 5 |
|---|---|---|---|---|---|
| 1. Quietness | – | | | | |
| 2. Self-expression | 0.146 | – | | | |
| 3. School adjustment | 0.345** | 0.186 | – | | |
| 4. Peer relations | 0.061 | 0.454** | 0.105 | – | |
| 5. Leaning engagement | 0.296* | 0.513** | 0.515** | 0.545** | – |
| 6. Academic performance | 0.241 | 0.063 | 0.317* | 0.026 | 0.067 |
| **CI in EA-dominant schools** | **1** | **2** | **3** | **4** | **5** |
| 1. Quietness | – | | | | |
| 2. Self-expression | −0.212 | – | | | |
| 3. School adjustment | −0.186 | 0.495** | – | | |
| 4. Peer relations | −0.520** | 0.421** | 0.394** | – | |
| 5. Learning engagement | −0.290* | 0.699** | 0.476** | 0.574** | – |
| 6. Academic performance | −0.182 | 0.253 | 0.142 | 0.506** | 0.303* |
| **EA children** | **1** | **2** | **3** | **4** | **5** |
| 1. Quietness | – | | | | |
| 2. Self-expression | −0.301* | – | | | |
| 3. School adjustment | 0.047 | 0.403** | – | | |
| 4. Peer relations | −0.097 | 0.307* | 0.116 | – | |
| 5. Learning engagement | 0.083 | 0.538** | 0.579** | 0.421* | – |
| 6. Academic performance | 0.150 | 0.034 | −0.202 | −0.366* | 0.013 |

\* $p < 0.05$, \*\* $p < 0.01$ (two tailed).
For analyses of CI children in Asian-dominant preschools and EA-dominant preschools, we controlled for SES. Since all EA children are middle-class, we did not control for SES.

assertion of one's own desires. As described earlier, CI children are likely to internalize a communication style that encourages them to be attentive and to listen to teachers rather than asserting their needs and opinions at school. To further disentangle the issues between teacher stereotypes and home and school contexts affecting CI children's quietness, future studies should examine differences in quietness and self-expression between home and school as well as gaps between mothers' and teachers' perceptions. Nevertheless, our findings are important since they present the reality of everyday school experiences among CI children, being quiet and less expressive or perceived to be so compared to their EA peers.

We found that the length of mothers' US residence as well as their SES were not related to CI children's verbal expression or quietness, indicating that cultural values regarding quietness and self-expression and their children's expression may be robust to parents' acculturation or social class positions. However, we found that the more proficient CI children were in English, the more expressive they were perceived in EA-dominant preschools, but not in Asian-dominant preschools. This finding is not surprising because CI children can speak their native language to communicate with their teachers and classmates in Chinese-dominant preschools. To communicate their needs and desires to American teachers, CI children must achieve a certain level of English proficiency. However, CI children's English proficiency was not related to their quietness, which was surprising. It is possible that quiet attitudes are deeply rooted in CI children's cultural values and norms, and cannot be easily changed through acquisition of language skills.[8] Still, this finding is consistent with the previous qualitative study which demonstrated Asian immigrant college students' quietness relative to EA students even when they obtained a high level of English proficiency [Liu, 2002]. Since differences in children's quietness and self-expression appear at this young age, we speculate that cultural values of quietness and non-assertiveness persist and are actively practiced in children's socialization among CI families [Cheah & Leung, 2011; Liu, in press].

*Consequences of Being Quiet*
Examination of two preschools with distinctive racial and cultural climates allowed us to study dissimilar school contexts in which quietness and self-expressions are positively or negatively rewarded. We found evidence showing different associations between children's quietness and school experiences, mainly in socioemotional and behavioral areas, that depended on the type of preschool attended by CI children. Quietness is associated with positive school experiences such as better school adjustment and better learning engagement if CI children attend an Asian-dominant preschool, but it is related to difficulties in peer relations and learning engagement if CI children attend an EA-dominant preschool. Interestingly, expressive and assertive children are likely to have more positive peer relations and learning engagement for both CI children and EA children regardless of types of school attended by them. Verbal expression was not related to children's academic performance, when SES was controlled. These results suggest that CI children's quietness may be associated with socioemotional development but not with their academic achievement. Even though more research is necessary to single out various factors underlying these associations, the basic findings of our research indicate that schools create environments that inhibit or promote cultural values shared by immigrant children [García Coll et al., 1996], and this practice may be associated with developmental outcomes.

These findings prompted us to raise the question: Are there any elements that mediate the association between quietness and/or self-expression on CI children's school and learning experiences? Unfortunately, our data do not allow us to test the mechanisms by which quietness affects children's preschool experiences positively or negatively in the two types of school. However, it would be useful to conjecture such mechanisms that can be explored and tested in future studies. Thus, we use our findings as a basis of our theoretical explorations, and propose three mediators through which quietness and self-expression can be rewarded differently in each school context: (a) teacher interactions, (b) peer acceptance, and (c) cultural continuity/discontinuity and children's acculturative stress.

Teacher Interactions
As Bronfenbrenner [1979] argued, the condition most immediate to children at preschool is their interaction with teachers and peers. Teachers' cultural expectations, especially when such expectations affect their day-to-day interactions with the child, create different school environments for immigrant children. Research has shown that teachers' views about the child

---

[8] It is also possible that CI children's temperament is associated with their quiet behaviors [Chen et al., 2009; Hart et al., 2000].

and home culture shape their engagement with the child [Kim, 2002; Lareau, 2003]. A study by Sirin, Ryce and Mir [2009] found that first grade teachers hold positive views toward students and families whose values are similar to theirs regardless of the parents' ethnicity. Teachers' ratings for students' academic competence and behavioral problems appear to be negative when teachers view children's parents as having discordant values. Most teachers in Asian-dominant preschools in our study are Asians, and they are likely to perceive quiet children positively – as mature, hardworking, and competent – since they are familiar with Asian culture. These teachers may even offer greater emotional support for quiet children to facilitate their school experiences and improve their relationships with their friends. Favorable interactions with their teachers are likely to facilitate positive school experiences of quiet children and their engagement in learning. In EA-dominant preschools, quiet children may become invisible [Archer & Francis, 2005], if not de-valued. Quiet children, in contrast to expressive children, may not stand out as an engaged learner or may even be viewed as a passive learner since EA cultures tend to associate verbal elaboration with competence and active thinking. This might explain negative association between quietness and learning engagement in EA-dominant preschools.

American teachers are likely to view expressive and assertive children as more competent and active learners. One early study that analyzed American teachers' views related to quietness and expressiveness documented that American teachers expected better class participation, academic performance, and peer relations for an expressive child than a quiet child [McCroskey & Daly, 1976]. When teachers hold positive perceptions about the students and their development, they are likely to provide more interactions and a more positive and challenging learning environment to these students [Weinstein, 2002]. It is possible that teachers provide more attention and support for expressive children, which facilitates these children's school adjustment. It is also possible that expressive children ask for more support from teachers.

Peer Acceptance
Reception by peers greatly influences children's school experiences, including their emotional, social, and cognitive development. Peers can become supportive or harmful for immigrant children's development depending on their response to the immigrant children's cultural backgrounds. A previous qualitative study demonstrated a high level of discrimination toward CI youth in the US [Qin et al., 2008]. Among adolescents, peer harassment of Asian Americans is severe [Rivas-Drake, Hughes & Way, 2008; Way, 1996]. Peer contexts in Asian-dominant preschools differ significantly from those in EA-dominant preschools. Our findings demonstrate that quiet CI children are less likely to get along with or less liked by peers in EA-dominant schools, but not in Asian-dominant preschools. Most children who attend Asian-dominant preschools are Asian and are likely to accept quiet children since their home culture encourages the development of positive views toward quietness. Moreover, teachers in Asian-dominant schools may try to create positive relationships between quiet children and their peers, which may reduce quiet children's negative relationships with peers. In addition, quietness is negatively associated with peer relations among CI children attending an EA-dominant preschool, but this relationship does not exist for EA children. We speculate that racial/ethnic difference might moderate this pathway. One empirical study has shown that most children have a concept of race and can identify people from different racial groups by preschool age [Aboud, 1988]. A different study found that EA children tend to demonstrate a stronger preference for same-race children than do minority children [Ramsey & Myers, 1990]. CI children may stand out as different from EA children when they are quiet in EA-dominant preschools. That is, quietness may

increase EA children's awareness of the racial/ethnic difference in CI children and may lead them to avoid quiet CI children. Our further analysis showed that ethnicity, merely being CI or EA, was not associated with negative peer relations in EA-dominant preschools. Thus, it could be the combination of being Asians and quiet that may be associated with negative relationships with their EA peers.

## Cultural Continuity/Discontinuity and Children's Acculturative Stress

When the cultural values at school create conflicts with the cultural values of home, immigrant children are likely to experience acculturative stress, which affects their behaviors, social relations, and learning engagement at school. Quiet children who attend Asian-dominant schools may find similar expectations for verbal expression at home and school. This cultural continuity between home and school is likely to reduce their acculturative stress, which leads to better school adjustment and positive attitudes toward learning at school. Quiet CI children attending an EA-dominant school may struggle between the two sets of norms regarding verbal expression: quietness had negative associations with these children's peer relations and learning engagement in EA-dominant preschools. But why do expressive CI children attending EA-dominant preschools fare better in school adjustment and learning engagement if quietness is encouraged in their home? Why is being expressive positive for CI children's learning engagement in Asian-dominant preschools, too? Some CI parents who are attuned to American norms may realize the value of verbal expression and assertiveness in American society and may incorporate these practices in their children's socialization processes. Moreover, teachers may encourage parents to facilitate their children's verbal expression at home, and the continuity between home and school may lead to better school adjustment and learning engagement for children. However, CI parents are not likely to discourage their children to be quiet when they encourage them to be expressive. CI parents are likely to view that quietness and expressiveness can coexist as we did not find negative correlations between quietness and self-expression among CI children as we did among EA children. CI children may become bicultural by internalizing the values related to communication styles at home and school, that is found to bring positive influence on immigrant children's psychological adaptations and academic trajectories [Fuligni, Witkow & Garcia, 2005; García Coll et al., 1996; Rumbaut, 1994]. However, major challenges are likely to appear when cultural norms at school and home are conflicting, and the children cannot cope with code switching.

## Conclusion: Developmental Indications

At age 4, we did not find a significant difference in teachers' ratings for children's school adjustment, peer relations, learning engagement, or academic outcomes between middle-class CI and EA children. Unlike studies on adolescents, children of middle-class CI families seem to be doing well or at least to the same extent as EA children during the preschool period in teachers' eyes. However, it is important to note that our assessment was rated by preschool teachers, which differs from most studies that rely on self-reports. Thus, we cannot conclude that CI children do not experience internal difficulties during the transition from home to school. Other types of assessment, such as observations, parent reports, and children's responses to hypothetical stories, are necessary to assess children's school adjustment more completely.

However, our findings warrant a theoretical shift from regarding quietness as a personality flaw compared to expressivity to a view that fluctuates depending on cultural values and contexts. Depending on the beholder, a quiet child may be perceived to be an inhibited communicator, possibly leading to reduced attention from teachers and peers, or a typical young child who needs nurturance, care, and encouragement from teachers and peers. We identified that CI children's quietness are associated with negative peer relations and lower engagement in learning in EA-dominant preschools, indicating that quietness and non-expressiveness are perhaps viewed as a cultural deficit in Western schools. These findings suggest the beginning of phenomena that can lead to greater difficulty for Asian immigrant children as their schooling continue, especially if they do not become bicultural. Due to negative views toward quietness and positive views toward self-expression in Western societies, Asian immigrant children are likely to face unforeseen challenges at school, including difficult school experiences and peer relations, unless they attend a school that has a significant number of Asian teachers or students. Because a high ratio of socioemotional problems has been reported among Asian American adolescents, we call for attention to this particular issue. As they grow older, other elements such as racial discrimination and prejudice may further interact with students' verbal expression and affect the pathways of Asian immigrant children regardless of SES.

Even though quietness was not related to children's academic performance at this age, we should not dismiss a possible association of quietness and academic performance at other ages, especially for low-SES CI children. A previous study found a large SES discrepancy in academic achievement within CI preschoolers [Li, Yamamoto, Luo, Batchelor & Bresnahan, 2010]. The present study identified that teacher ratings for learning engagement in addition to academic performance among low-SES children were significantly lower than those for middle-class CI children. Most low-SES CI children in the present study attended Asian-dominant preschools. Some of the low-SES CI children may continue to attend a school with a high ratio of Asian teachers and students since they tend to live in ethnic enclaves such as Chinatowns. However, when low-SES children attend an EA-dominant school, quiet children may become at risk of falling behind since they may not elicit the attention and support needed from their teachers to advance their academic development. As recent research has demonstrated, teacher involvement and support are more powerful in affecting low-SES students' academic processes than those of middle-class students [Benner & Mistry, 2007; Weinstein, 2002].

The number of Asian American children has doubled to represent 4.2% of the total student population in the US. Despite the sharp increase in Asian populations in American classrooms, Asian teachers are underrepresented in American schools; they represent only 1.2% of all K-12 teachers [National Center for Education Statistics, 2008]. Most teachers in the US are EA and have limited experience with Asian American children [Goodwin, 2002]. In addition to exerting greater effort to recruit Asian American teachers, it is critical to ensure that all teachers are aware of their negative perceptions of quietness and the associated potential neglect of quiet children that can lead to difficulty in adaptations to the school processes [McCoskey, 1980]. Increasing teachers' understanding of various communication styles among immigrant children and their families, teachers' efforts to facilitate peer relationships between quiet children and others, and their efforts to understand quiet children's needs might help ease Asian immigrant children's adjustment to school.

Before concluding, it is important to note several limitations in our study. Firstly, the current study relied on teacher ratings for assessment of children's verbal expression. Thus, we cannot determine if CI children are actually quiet and less expressive at school or are perceived to be so by teachers. Other types of assessment are critical to evaluate children's verbal expression more completely. Secondly, participants of our study were recruited from two states in the Northeastern part of the US. Therefore, our findings may not be generalizable to CI children in other states or countries. Future studies which examine school and social contexts surrounding Asian immigrant children in other states and other Western countries would extend our understandings about social attitudes toward quietness and Asian immigrant children's experiences depending on contexts. Lastly, even though we discussed about quietness and self-expression in East Asian immigrant contexts, we focused on Chinese immigrants in the present study. It is critical to investigate other ethnic groups such as Japanese, Korean, and other Asian immigrant children in order to further test our theory.

As stated earlier, not enough attention has been paid to the relationship between verbal expression and the development of Asian immigrant children in Western school contexts. Our study has begun to open up this line of research. We look forward to more research that adopts the sociocultural and contextual framework. Such a theoretical shift may allow us to generate more valid research which empirically examines important moderators and mediators of verbal expression that impact Asian immigrant children's development in their host countries.

## Appendix

*Learning Engagement Items*
How is the child's attitude and behavior towards learning?
1 = Rarely applies, 2 = Sometimes applies, 3 = Average, 4 = Usually applies, 5 = Always applies.
1. Is bored with learning activities.
2. Explores new activities on own.
3. Does not pay attention.
4. Takes initiative.
5. Likes to come to school.
6. Uninterested in/does not enjoy learning.
7. Eager to do well.
8. Is creative in learning.
9. Does not listen to teacher.
10. Unable to concentrate.
11. Can face setbacks.
12. Does not ask questions.
13. Has fun doing learning activities at school.
14. Relies heavily on others during learning activities.
15. Does not take responsibility for self.
16. Is discouraged in the face of failure.
17. Follows teacher's directions.
18. Fails to try/give effort.
19. Does not respect teacher.
20. Always wants to learn more.
21. Wants to try new things.
22. Does not finish the given activity.
23. Gives continuous effort.
24. Is cooperative with authority figures.
25. Does not finish task once interrupted.
26. Participates willingly in learning activities.
27. Gives up easily.
28. Does not care about achievement in learning.
29. Wants to improve (self).

## Acknowledgements

This research was supported by grants awarded to Jin Li from the Foundation for Child Development and the Spencer Foundation. The authors thank Lily Luo, Jia Li Liu, Yuhong Huang, Helen Pang, Caroline Segal, and other students for their assistance with data collection. The authors are grateful to Charissa S. L. Cheah and Cindy H. Liu for their advice. Special thanks go to children and parents and many daycare centers, schools, and organizations that made this study possible.

## References

Aboud, F.E. (1988). *Children and prejudice*. New York: Blackwell.

Alegria, M. (2009). The challenge of acculturation measures: What are we missing? A commentary on Thomson & Hoffman-Goetz. *Social Science & Medicine, 69*, 996–998.

Archer, L., & Francis, B. (2005). 'They never go off the rails like other ethnic groups': Teachers' constructions of British Chinese pupils' gender identities and approaches to learning. *British Journal of Sociology of Education, 26*, 165–182.

Azuma, H. (1986). Why study child development in Japan? In H. Stevenson, H. Azuma & K. Hakuta (Eds.), *Child development and education in Japan and the United States* (pp. 147–166). New York: Freeman.

Bankston, C.L., & Zhou, M. (2002). Social-emotional factors affecting achievement outcomes among disadvantaged students: Closing the achievement gap. *Educational Psychologist, 37*, 197–214.

Barnett, S.W., Epstein, D.J., Friedman, A.H., Sansanelli, R.A., & Hustedt, J.T. (2009). *The state of preschool: 2009 state preschool yearbook.* New Brunswick: National Institute for Early Education Research (NIEER).

Benner, A.D., & Mistry, R.S. (2007). Congruence of mother and teacher educational expectations and low-income youth's academic competence. *Journal of Educational Psychology, 99*, 140–153.

Bronfenbrenner, U. (1979). *The ecology of human development: Experiments by nature and design.* Cambridge, MA: Harvard University Press.

Caudill, W., & Weinstein, H. (1969). Maternal care and infant behavior in Japan and America. *Psychiatry, 32*, 12–43.

Cheah, C.S.L., & Leung, C.Y.Y., (2011). The social development of immigrant children: A focus on Asian and Hispanic children in the U.S. In P.K. Smith & C.H. Hart (Eds.), *Wiley-Blackwell handbook of childhood social development* (pp. 225–241). Wiley-Blackwell Publishers.

Chen, X., Chen, H., Li, D., & Wang, L. (2009). Early childhood behavioral inhibition and social and school adjustment in Chinese children: A 5-year longitudinal study. *Child Development, 80*, 1692–1704.

Chen, X., Hastings, P.D., Rubin, K.H., Chen, H., Cen, G., & Stewart, S. (1998). Child-rearing attitudes and behavioral inhibition in Chinese and Canadian toddlers: A cross-cultural study. *Developmental Psychology, 34*, 677–686.

Chen, X., Rubin, K.H., & Li, Z. (1995). Social functioning and adjustment in Chinese children: A longitudinal study. *Developmental Psychology, 31*, 531–539.

Davies, R.J., & Ikeno, O. (2002). *The Japanese mind: Understanding contemporary Japanese culture.* Rutland: Tuttle Publishing

Duncan, S., & De Avila, E. (1998). *Pre-LAS 2000.* Monterey: McGraw-Hill.

Fuligni, A.J., Witkow, M., & Garcia, C. (2005). Ethnic identity and the academic adjustment of adolescents from Mexican, Chinese, and European backgrounds. *Developmental Psychology, 41*, 799–811.

García Coll, C.T., Lamberty, G., Jenkins, R., McAdoo, H.P., Crnic, K., Wasik, B.H., & Vazquez García, H. (1996). An integrative model for the study of developmental competencies in minority children. *Child Development, 67*, 1891–1914.

García Coll, C.T., & Marks, A. (2009). *Immigrant stories: Ethnicity and academics in middle childhood.* New York, NY: Oxford University Press.

Goodwin, A.L. (2002). Teacher preparation and the education of immigrant children. *Education and Urban Society, 34*, 156–172.

Hao, L., & Bonstead-Bruns, M. (1998). Parent-child differences in educational expectations and the academic achievement of immigrant and native students. *Sociology of Education, 71*, 175–198.

Hart, C.H., Yang, C., Nelson, L.J., Robinson, C.C., Olsen, J.A., Nelson, D.A., Porter, C.L., Jin, S., Olsen, S.F., & Wu, P. (2000). Peer acceptance in early childhood and subtypes of socially withdrawn behaviour in China, Russia, and the United States. *International Journal of Behavioral Development, 24*, 73–81.

Hollingshead, A.B. (1975). Four-factor index of social status. Unpublished manuscript, Yale University.

Holloway, S.D. (2010). *Women and family in contemporary Japan.* New York: Cambridge University Press.

Holloway, S.D., & Yamamoto, Y. (2003). Sensei! Early childhood education teachers in Japan. In O. Saracho & B. Spodek (Eds.), *Contemporary perspectives in early childhood education: Studying teachers in early childhood setting* (pp. 181–207). Greenwich: Information Age Publishing.

Inagaki, K., Hatano, G., & Morita, E. (1998). Construction of mathematical knowledge through whole-class discussion. *Learning and Instruction, 8,* 503–526.

Ishii, S., & Bruneau, T. (1994). Silence and silences in cross-cultural perspective: Japan and the United States. In L.A. Samovar & R.E. Porter (Eds.), *Intercultural communication: A reader* (7th ed., pp. 246–251). Belmont: Wadsworth.

Kao, G. (1995). Asian Americans as model minorities? A look at their academic performance. *American Journal of Education, 103*, 121–159.

Kao, G. (1999). Psychological well-being and educational achievement among immigrant youth. *International Migration Review, 38*, 427–449.

Kim, A., & Yeh, C.J. (2002). *Stereotype of Asian American students. ERIC Digest.* Retrieved from ERIC database (ED462510).

Kim, H.S. (2002). We talk, therefore, we think? A cultural analysis of the effect of talking on thinking. *Journal of Personality and Social Psychology, 83*, 828–842.

Lareau, A. (2003). *Unequal childhoods: Class, race and family life.* Berkeley: University of California Press.

Lebra, T.S. (1976). *Japanese patterns of behavior.* Honolulu: The University Press of Hawaii.

Lebra, T.S. (1987). The cultural significance of silence in Japanese communication. *Multilingua, 6*, 343–357.

Lei, J.L. (2003). (Un)Necessary toughness?: Those 'loud black girls' and those 'quiet Asian boys.' *Anthropology & Education Quarterly, 34*, 158–181.

Li, G., & Wang, L. (2008). *Model minority myth revisited: An interdisciplinary approach to demystifying Asian American educational experiences.* Charlotte: Information Age Publishing.

Li, J. (in press). *Cultural foundations of learning: East and West.* New York: Cambridge University Press.

Li, J., & Sklar, S. (2010). To speak or not to speak: European American eagerness versus Chinese reluctance. Manuscript in preparation.

Li, J., Yamamoto, Y., Luo, L., Batchelor, A., & Bresnahan, R. (2010). Why attend school? Chinese immigrant and European American preschoolers' views and outcomes. *Developmental Psychology, 46*, 1637–1650.

Liu, C.H. (2011). Emotion development in Asian American youth and children. In F. Leong, L. Juang, D.B. Qin & H.E. Fitzgerald (Eds.), *Asian American and pacific islander children and mental health. Vol. 1* (pp. 97–120). New York: Praeger Press.

Liu, J. (2002). Negotiating silence in American classrooms: Three Chinese cases. *Language and intercultural communication, 2*, 37–54.

Marks, A.K., Patton, F., & García Coll, C. (2010). More than the A-B-Cs and 1–2–3s: The importance of family cultural socialization and ethnic identity development for children of immigrants' early school success. In E.L. Grigorenko & R. Takanishi (Eds.), *Immigration, diversity, and education* (pp. 242–258). New York: Routledge.

Markus, H.R., & Kitayama, S. (1991). Culture and the self: Implications for cognition, emotion, and motivation. *Psychological Review, 98,* 224–253.

Mathews, R. (2000). Cultural patterns of South Asian and Southeast Asian Americans. *Intervention in School and Clinic, 36,* 101–104.

McCroskey, J.C. (1980). Quiet children in the classroom: On helping not hurting. *Communication Education, 29,* 239–244.

McCroskey, J.C., & Daly, J. (1976). Teachers' expectations of the communication apprehensive child in the elementary school. *Human Communication Research, 3,* 67–72.

Miller, P.J., Fung, H., Lin. S.-M., Chen, E.C.-H., & Boldt, B.R. (in press). *Personal storytelling as a socializing practice in Taiwanese and European-American families: A longitudinal study of alternate developmental pathways. Monographs of the Society for Research in Child Development.*

Minami, M. (1994). English and Japanese: A cross-cultural comparison of parental styles of narrative elicitation. *Issues in Applied Linguistics, 5,* 383–407.

Minami, M., & McCabe, A. (1995). Rice balls and bear hunts: Japanese and North American family narrative patterns. *Journal of Child Language, 22,* 423–445.

Murase, T., Dale, P.S., Ogura, T., Yamashita, Y., & Mahieu, A. (2005). Mother-child conversation during joint picture book reading in Japan and the USA. *First Language, 25,* 197–218.

National Center for Education Statistics (2008). Number and percentage distribution of public elementary and secondary school teachers, by locale and selected characteristics: 2007–08. http://nces.ed.gov/surveys/ruraled/tables/c.1.a.-1.asp?refer=urban

Ng, J.C., Lee, S.S., & Pak, Y.K. (2007). Contesting the model minority and perpetual foreigner stereotypes: A critical review of literature on Asian Americans in education. *Review of Research in Education, 31,* 95–130.

Qin, D.B., Way, N., & Mukherjee, P. (2008). The other side of the model minority story: The familial and peer challenges face by Chinese American adolescents. *Youth & Society, 39,* 480–506.

Ramsey, P.G., & Myers, L.C. (1990) Salience of race in young children's cognitive, affective, and behavioral responses to social environments. *Journal of Applied Developmental Psychology, 11,* 49–67.

Remedios, L., Clarke, D.J., & Hawthorne, L. (2008). The silent participant in small group collaborative learning contexts. *Active Learning in Higher Education, 9,* 201–216.

Rivas-Drake, D., Hughes, D., & Way, N. (2008). A closer look at peer discrimination, ethnic identity, and psychological well-being among urban Chinese American sixth graders. *Journal Youth Adolescence, 37,* 12–21.

Rubin, K.H., & Mills, R.S. (1988). The many faces of social isolation in childhood. *Journal of Consulting and Clinical Psychology, 56,* 916–924.

Rumbaut, R.G. (1994). The crucible within: Ethnic identity, self-esteem, and segmented assimilation among children of immigrants. *International Migration Review, 28,* 748–781.

Sirin, S.R., Ryce, P., & Mir, M. (2009). How teachers' values affect their evaluation of children of immigrants. *Early Childhood Research Quarterly, 24,* 463–473.

Suárez-Orozco, C., Suárez-Orozco, M.M., & Todorova, I. (2008). *Learning a new land: Immigrant students in American society.* Cambridge: Harvard University Press.

Sy, S.R., & Schulenberg, J.E. (2005). Parent beliefs and children's achievement trajectories during the transition to school in Asian American and European American families. *International Journal of Behavioral Development, 29,* 505–515.

Takeishi, C.A. (2008). Taking a chance with words. *Rethinking Schools, 22,* 20–23. Retrieved on December 16, 2010, http://www.rethinkingschools.org/restrict.asp?path=archive/22_02/word222.shtml.

Tannen, D., & Saville-Troike, M. (1985). *Perspectives on silence.* Norwood: Ablex Publishing Corporation.

US Census Bureau. (2007). *Minority populations tops 100 million* (Release No. CB07–70). http://www.census.gov/newsroom/releases/archives/population/cb07–70.html.

US Census Bureau. (2011). Overview of race and Hispanic origin: 2010 (Release No. C2010BR-02). http://www.census.gov/prod/cen2010/briefs/c2010br-02.pdf.

Way, N. (1996). Between experiences of betrayal and desire: Close friendships among urban adolescents. In B. J. Leadbeater & N. Way (Eds.), *Urban girls: Resisting stereotypes, creating identities* (pp. 173–192). New York: New York University Press.

Weinstein, R. (2002). *Reaching higher: The power of expectations in schooling.* Cambridge, MA: Harvard University Press.

Yamamoto, Y., & Holloway, S.D. (2010). Parental expectations and children's academic performance in sociocultural contexts. *Educational Psychology Review, 22,* 189–214.

Zhou, M., & Kim, R. (2006). The paradox of ethnicization and assimilation: The development of ethnic organizations in the Chinese immigrant community in the United States. In K.E. Kuah-Pearce & E. Hu-Dehart (Eds.), *Voluntary organizations in the Chinese diaspora* (pp. 231–252). Hong Kong: Hong Kong University Press.

Yoko Yamamoto
Department of Education, Brown University
Providence, RI 02912 (USA)
E-Mail Yoko_Yamamoto@brown.edu

# The Impact of Social Contexts in Schools: Adolescents Who Are New to Canada and Their Sense of Belonging

Monique H. Gagné · Jennifer D. Shapka · Danielle M. Law

Department of Education and Counseling Psychology and Special Education, University of British Columbia, Vancouver, B.C., Canada

## Abstract

Young people are breaking many of the preconceived notions we have about the immigration experience and its impact on development. Consistent with an emerging pattern in a number of host countries, new young Canadians are emerging with positive outcomes on a number of developmental outcomes, including academic, psychosocial, and health. Moving forward, researchers are delving deeper and expanding their notion of 'success' for young newcomers and finding a powerful mediator to these positive outcomes: social support. As such, this chapter focuses on the social life of young newcomers at school, and includes discussion of a study which investigated how school social context (various types of social support, school diversity, perceived racial/ethnic and linguistic similarity) impact perceptions of school belonging for adolescents who are new to Canada (as compared with non-newcomers). Using a sample of 733 adolescents (grades 5–12), from public schools in the Lower Mainland of British Columbia, hierarchical regression analyses indicated that perceived racial/ethnic and linguistic similarity to other students at school, adult support for school and personal help, and peer support for 'hanging out' were associated with school belonging for adolescents who were new to Canada. In addition, moderator analysis revealed that newer generation Canadians were impacted differently by social support at school. That is, they had a stronger relationship between adult support for school help and school belonging, as well as with peer support for personal help and school belonging.

Copyright © 2012 S. Karger AG, Basel

These are unprecedented times of migration throughout the world, with Canada being no exception. In fact, Canada has one of the highest rates of immigration in the world with 18.9% of the total population being foreign-born [Berry, Westin, Virta, Vedder, Rooney & Sang, 2006]. For young newcomers to Canada, schools will be where they spend the vast majority of their time. As such, school contexts will play a determining factor in a newcomer's successful adaptation to a new country. In a summary of the G8 Report on diversity and integration, the impact of school systems on the various needs of young newcomers to Canada was highlighted and emphasized [Citizenship and Immigration Canada, 2006]. Obviously, academic success is an important component of successful adaptation, but schools have much more to offer newcomers than simply an avenue for attaining positive academic outcomes. They have the potential to provide foundations for positive social and emotional development by offering newcomers salient knowledge, social connections, and ultimately, a sense of belonging in their new home.

In comparison to academics, far less is known about how these children and adolescents are emotionally adapting at school. We know that having a sense of school belonging – defined as 'the extent to which students feel personally accepted, respected, included and supported by others in the school social environment' [Goodenow, 1993, p. 80] – helps satisfy an individual's social needs [Watson, Battistich & Solomon, 1997]. In fact, in general, the importance of school context on social and emotional needs has begun to garner increasing amounts of research attention [Hymel, Schonert-Reichl & Miller, 2007], but there is a lack of research that considers how the social factors present in a school context might uniquely impact the sense of school belonging for those who have recently immigrated. This is despite the fact that there is evidence which indicates that school contexts can impact children differently based on factors such as immigration status, minority status, and socioeconomic status (SES) [Garcia Coll and Marks, 2009; Garcia Coll, in press; Han, 2008; Suarez-Orozco & Suarez-Orozco, 2001]. This chapter intends to address the role of school context for newcomers to Canada, first by providing an overview of the social life of immigrants at school and then by describing a study which focused on the extent to which adolescents who are new to Canada feel a sense of belonging at school.

**The Immigrant Paradox**

For newcomers, the factors that would typically imply 'risk' are abundant. Those who immigrate are thought to undergo acculturative stress, in response to the psychological stressors from adapting to a new culture and learning a new language [Hernandez, 2009]. This can be compounded by experiences of racism and discrimination [Suarez-Orozco & Suarez-Orozco, 2001]. In addition, immigrants tend to be poorer and have less social and economic capital [Beiser, Hou, Hyman & Tousignant, 2002; Hernandez, 2004]. They are also more likely to attend large inner-city schools and have less knowledge as to how the school system works [Garcia Coll & Marks, 2009]. Intuitively and theoretically, this level of exposure to such a multitude of risk factors would suggest initially those who immigrate should show signs of struggle, given the increased challenges they are facing, but over time, they would adapt, which would be reflected by positive health, behavioral, and academic outcomes.

In reality however, the outcomes reported for those who immigrate are more variable than what might be predicted given our traditional notions of what it means to be 'at risk'. There is mounting evidence that some young immigrants are demonstrating academic success that is on par with and oftentimes better than their non-immigrant counterparts even after taking into account the multitude of challenges they can face. This pattern has been illustrated in numerous studies in both the US [Fuligni, 1997; Garcia Coll & Marks, 2009; Garcia Coll, in press; Kao & Tienda, 1995] and in Canada [Beiser, Hou, Hyman & Tousignant, 1998; McAndrew et al., 2009]. There is also mounting evidence to indicate that they are generally physically healthier and engage in less risky behaviors [Chen, Ng & Wilkins, 1996; McDonald & Kennedy, 2004; Perez, 2002; Garcia Coll & Marks, 2009; Garcia Coll & Marks, in press]. As research accumulates against traditional models of adaptation, scholars have articulated a new pattern of developmental trajectories – often termed the *Immigrant Paradox*. Despite these emerging patterns, the pathways of adaptation for young people who immigrate are far from uniform [Fuligni 1997; Kao & Tienda, 1995; McAndrew et al., 2009; Portes & Rumbaut, 2001], and they can mask important inter-group differences [McAndrew et al., 2009; Suarez-Orozco et al., 2010] – making it necessary to shift the focus toward understanding the subtleties that may contribute to both individual and group differences.

Patterns of emotional adaptation for young people who immigrate seem to be particularly varied and in need of investigation. There are mixed findings regarding the well-being of newly immigrated youth [Fuligni, 1998; Takeuchi, Hong, Gile & Alegria, 2007]. There are some findings to indicate positive mental health outcomes for newcomers [Crosnoe, 2006; Hough et al., 2002]. In fact, reports from Canada, New Zealand, Europe, and the US suggest that first-generation immigrants fare more positively on a number of indicators of well-being in comparison to their peers who are native-born [Suarez-Orozco & Carhill, 2008]. In addition to these findings however, others have found no mental health and psychopathology differences between immigrants and non-immigrants [Alegria, Sribney, Woo, Torres & Guarnaccia, 2007; Suarez-Orozco & Qin-Hilliard, 2004]. For example, immigration status does not predict self-esteem or positive psychological well-being [Fuligni, 1998]. To add to the complexity, there have also been some less than positive findings. For instance, young immigrants tend to perceive less control over their lives and feel less popular than their native-born peers [Chiu, Feldman & Rosenthal, 1992; Kao, 1999]. Clearly, more work is needed to explore the robustness of the immigrant paradox across emotional domains.

Fortunately, the idea that we need to pay heed to the social and emotional needs and status of adolescents from immigrant backgrounds in schools is gaining momentum and empirical support [Hymel et al., 2007]. This focus can be partly attributed to the scientific base connecting social and emotional learning to school success [Zins, Bloodworth, Weissberg & Walberg, 2004]. Students are more apt to learn and be academically successful when they perceive that their school values them and cares about them [Elias, 2006].

There are a number of factors of school social contexts that might impact one's experience with school for those who immigrate: First, they may perceive different amounts of support from the peers and adults at their school. Second, they may attend schools that have cultural compositions in which they feel similar or different from others. It is critical to establish the extent to which these social factors at school may help to meet the emotional needs of young people who immigrate. In borrowing the words from Claude Steele, 'It is one thing to integrate a school setting or work place. It is another thing to make that setting a place where they feel like they belong' [National Research Council, 2007, p. 3]. The study described in this chapter will add to our understanding of this question by exploring how factors of the school social context impact the perceived sense of belonging to school for immigrant vs. non-immigrant youth.

**Belonging**

Belonging to a community is frequently considered the foundation for learning and emotional support [Anderman & Freeman, 2004; Baumeister & Leary, 1995; Maehr & Midgley, 1996; Osterman, 2000; Rogoff, 1990]. Evidence suggests that students function better when they feel that they belong to their school context [Ryan, 1995]. Specifically, belongingness has been linked to a broad range of positive emotions such as happiness, contentment, and calm, all of which have positive implications for the overall socioemotional growth of an individual [Osterman, 2000]. Conversely, rejection by peers at school is associated with far-reaching adjustment problems, such as low self-esteem, anxiety, depression, criminal behavior, and early school withdrawal [McDougall, Hymel, Vaillancourt & Mercer, 2001].

The need for a sense of belonging to schools and receipt of necessary supports at school may vary depending on the student and the context within which they find themselves [Osterman, 2000]. This is in a similar vein to Eccles and Midgley's [1989] 'Stage-environment fit' theory, which suggests that different children at different developmental stages will benefit from different educational environments. For example, we know that adolescents tend to be more vulnerable to feelings of isolation than children [Certo, Cauley & Chafin, 2003; Osterman, 2000]. Furthermore, adolescents are especially prone to school maladjustment if they are in the midst of a significant period of stress [Eccles & Midgley, 1989]. This premise may be applicable to newcomers, who need to adjust to a new school, especially if their school environment is not conducive to fostering their own optimal development.

Social psychological literature suggests that the ways in which young people see themselves as part of a larger context, such as schools, is heavily influenced by the ways in which they interact with their social context [Sonderegger, Barrett & Creed, 2004]. This literature generally purports that amidst cultural transitions, social support is positively related to psychological well-being at school [Coleman, 1961; Sonderegger et al., 2004]. However, there have been few research contributions in the area of social support at school for new young Canadians.

**School Social Context**

The current study will add to this literature by looking at factors of the school social context that may help to explain feelings of school belonging across generations of immigrants. One aspect is the composition of a school, meaning the extent to which students feel similar to the rest of the student body. A second point of interest is the extent to which students feel they have support from people at school, from both peers and adults.

*Perceived Similarity*
*Racial/Ethnic Background.* Countless studies have examined the dynamics of race, ethnicity, and children. Yet, our knowledge in this area remains far from complete [Onyekwuluje, 1998]. Teasing apart racial/ethnic background and immigration status is becoming more of a priority as it becomes clear that they may operate differently in child development outcomes [Quintana et al., 2006]. In both Canadian and American contexts, there is evidence suggesting that ethnic and racial perceptions are highly influential in friendship choices for both first and second generation immigrants [Phan, 2003; Quillian & Campbell, 2003].

*Language.* Language also plays a large role in friendship formations: Individuals who cannot speak the language of the majority find it difficult to form friendships and social networks [Tsai, 2006]. Research also suggests that language ability for adolescents who have immigrated is a salient aspect of their social relationship choices at school. For example, those who have immigrated have been found to suffer from a fear of embarrassment and/or harassment by non-immigrant peers if they have not yet mastered the dominant language [Tsai, 2006]. As such, it has been theorized that children who immigrate choose friends who can speak their native language and avoid those who do not, in an attempt to protect their psychological well-being [Tatum, 1999]. These choices have significant repercussions for other developmental tasks such as identity and belonging, as well as cultural capital on how to succeed in school [Bailey, 2001; Kiang & Fuligni, 2009].

Taken together, the extent to which a young person speaks the same languages and comes from the same racial/ethnic background as others at school, might provide us with a sense of how culturally similar those who immigrate feel to others in their school environment. This notion of perceived similarity has been shown to influence a sense of belonging at school. Adolescence is a time when individuals become more exclusive in their friendship formations. Adolescents have a tendency to form friendships based on perceived similarities with others [Bellmore, Nishina, Graham & Juvonen, 2007; Bernt, 1981; Graham & Cohen, 1997]. This pattern of friendship formation has been shown to be moderated by factors such as a child's social milieu, their cultural status, and the level of contact they have with people who they perceive as different from themselves [Rotheram & Phinney, 1987]. The direction of impact that similarity may have on a student's sense of school belonging can be informed by research on ethnic enclaves. Living in an ethnic enclave can be associated with negative consequences such as isolation and missed opportunities for cultural capital [Garcia Coll & Marks, 2009]. In contrast, there is evidence to suggest that ethnic enclaves can also offer benefits such as support thereby fostering both academic and social development in young people [Garcia Coll et al., 1996; Garcia Coll & Marks, 2009; Portes, 2000].

*Social Support*
Adolescents who immigrate are faced with the challenge of leaving their friendships and social networks behind and making new connections in a new country [Tsai, 2006]. A major advantage of attending school is that it is an environment that is amenable to building friendships and social networks, thereby allowing youth to gain information about the new culture that they have been immersed into [Raffo & Reeves, 2000]. Unfortunately, the research that has been conducted in this area has been criticized for its narrow view of social support [Chen, 2001]. This critique is often extended to mention the lack of differentiation between type and quality of social support [Chen, 2001]. In addition to these critiques, it has been suggested that the literature rarely takes into account the larger social context of the school [Tsai, 2006].

It is argued that these weak findings are a result of previous studies limiting the interest of social interaction at school to specific dyadic 'best' friend types of relationships rather than to the broader context of peer groups and networks [Chen, 2001]. Indeed, it has been argued that the source of social support (i.e. peer, teacher, and family), as well as the type of social support (i.e. emotional, instructional, and companionship) must be distinguished in order to understand the pattern of influence [Wenz-Gross, Siperstein, Untch & Widaman, 1997]. Given that the function of social ties can vary tremendously, it is important to account for the different possible functions of school social support, specifically, school help (i.e. helping with homework), personal help (i.e. asking for help because of feelings of sadness, anger, or stress), and companionship or 'hanging out' (i.e. having lunch together, playing sports) and its relationship to the socioemotional development of new young Canadians.

*Peer Social Support*
Peer groups and social networks have long been venerated by theorists and researchers as influential in child development [Piaget, 1932; Sullivan, 1953]. They are thought to be key in dealing with emotional stressors and adjustment [Rubin, Bukowski, Parker, 1998]. There is a large body of research to suggest that students tend to view school more favorably and perform better at school when they are accepted by their peers [Ladd, 1990] and peers have an especially important role to play in the reception of newcomers [Yoshikawa & Way, 2008]. Coupled with these findings is research that suggests that intimate friendships at school are key to psychologically bonding to schools and in turn, feeling a sense of school belonging [Ryan, 2001].

*Adult/Teacher Social Support*
In the context of the school, it has been established that the role of the teacher is important to students, not only academically, but also socially and emotionally [Furman & Buhrmester, 1992]. Previous research has shown that perceived teacher support is even more important for adolescents who have immigrated than for adolescents who are native to that country. In a study conducted in the Netherlands, researchers found that adolescents who had immigrated placed a larger emphasis on teacher support, both instructionally and emotionally, than did students who were native to the country [Vedder, Boekarts & Seegers, 2005].

## The Current Study

To summarize, there are a number of factors that may impact a young person's sense of school belonging. Racial/ethnic background, Generation status, and Years in Canada will be used as markers of immigration experiences and how that may impact levels of School belonging. The first dimension of school social context, Perceived similarity, will function to represent a subjective measure of the cultural composition of the school. The second dimension of school social context considered here are five types of perceived social support at school: Adult support for school, Adult support for personal help, Peer support for school help, Peer support for personal help, and Peer support for hanging out. The current study was undertaken not only to determine how newcomers to Canada are faring in this regard, but also to identify how this may be moderated by Generation status. Essentially, this study goes beyond a main effects model in determining the causes and correlates of School belonging by considering Generation status as a moderator of the school social context variables.

Using data drawn from a large, multiethnic urban centre on the west coast of Canada, three research questions guided this study: (1) Are length of time in Canada, generation status, and racial/ethnic background associated with students' sense of school belonging? (2) In what ways are perceptions of school social context associated with school belonging? (3) Is the relationship between school social support and school belonging moderated by generation status?

## Method

*Participants*
Participants (n = 733) were recruited from grade 5 through 12 classes from six secondary (71% of the sample) and two elementary schools in the Lower mainland of British Columbia. Participants were asked to complete a questionnaire during class time which asked them demographic information, their racial/ethnic background, generational status, perceived racial/ethnic and language similarity, adult and peer social support at school, and sense of school belonging. All participants who consented (49% response rate) were included in the study, regardless of their generation status. Sixty-two percent of the sample was female[1], and the mean age of the sample was 15 years. Thirty percent of the sample indicated that they were from a single parent family (which was used as a proxy to represent SES[2]. Regarding ethnicity, 45.7% of the sample reported being of Asian descent, 33.7% of European descent, and 17.6% were incorporated into an 'other' category. The Other ethnicity category was a heterogeneous group (comprised of small groups of Aboriginal, African/Caribbean, South Asian, Latin American, Middle Eastern, and Mixed descent) and was created to preserve statistical power in our analyses.

*Measures*
*Gender, Grade, and Lone Parenting.* These demographic variables were entered as covariates in the model to account for any gender, developmental, and socioeconomic differences, respectively. Gender and Lone parenting were dummy-coded such that females and participants from single-parent families were coded as 1.

*Racial/Ethnic Background.* Participants were asked to choose their racial/ethnic background from a list of choices and examples to go along with each choice. Although it is recognized that *race* and *ethnicity* are generally distinguished between in the literature, it was not assumed that adolescents also make this distinction. The overwhelming majority of participants identified themselves as of Asian or European descent. All of the other racial/ethnic groupings were very small. Nevertheless, they were entered into the analysis as separate variables until it was clear that they had no impact on the outcome of the model. Finally, to preserve power, all of the ethnicities represented by small numbers of individuals were incorporated into the Other ethnicity category. This group was composed of Aboriginal, African/Caribbean, South Asian, Latin American, Middle Eastern, and Mixed variables. The groups compiled in the Other ethnicity category had group sizes that ranged from 6 to 55. Some participants (3%) chose 'I don't know' in response to this question, and those responses were coded as missing. Dummy variables were created for those of European descent and of Other

---

[1] The unbalanced gender split in the sample was due to data collection in several all-girls classes. The effect of this variable was controlled for in all statistical analyses.
[2] Although we originally aimed to use mothers' and fathers' education variable to assess SES, we had to use single parenting variable as a proxy due to large amount of missing data for education variables (50% of the sample reported that they did not know their parents' education level).

descent, and in all analyses, the reference group was Asian because it represented the largest racial/ethnic group in the sample.

*Generational Status.* Students were asked to answer questions about where they were born and where their parents were born in order to determine their generation status. From these questions, a Generational status variable was created using Rumbaut's [2008] classification scheme. This scheme categorizes participants as 1.5, 2nd, or 3rd generation Canadian. 1.5 generational status refers to a person who is foreign born, but arrived as a child or adolescent. A person labeled as 2nd generation Canadian was born in Canada, but at least one parent was foreign born. Finally, 3rd generation Canadian refers to any person who was born in Canada and has parents that were born in Canada. For the current study, 19.2% of the participants were 1.5 generation immigrants, 48.2% were 2nd generation immigrants, and 32.6% were 3rd generation or more. The age of the participants was distributed fairly evenly, with the mean age of 1.5, 2nd, and 3rd generation groups of 14.96, 14.47, and 15.32, respectively. Generational differences were more apparent in terms of the racial/ethnic background of participants. 1st generation and 2nd generation participants were most likely to be of Asian descent (accounting for 74.8 and 63.6% of the groups, respectively), and in contrast, 3rd generation participants were most likely to be of European descent (accounting for 72.8% of the group).

*Years in Canada.* In order to account for the length of time that a first generation adolescent has lived in Canada, a 'Years in Canada' variable was created. This variable was created to capture the subtle differences in the length of time adolescents have been in Canada (and in particular those with 1.5 Generation status). It ranged from under 1 year in Canada to 16 years in Canada, with the average newcomer living in Canada for 6.88 years. It was expected that this variable would be significantly correlated with Generation status. With a significant correlation of 0.60, both tolerance and VIF collinearity diagnostics ensured multicollinearity was not an issue.

*School Social Context*

*Perceived School Similarity.* Students' perceptions of how similar their peers at school are to themselves were assessed on a Likert scale, ranging from 1 'none of them' to 5 'all of them'. A sixth point was reserved for an 'I don't know' alternative response. A composite variable was created to capture each student's overall perception of similarity with the other students at their school by calculating the mean scores of both racial/ethnic and language similarity variables. Items which asked how similar students feel to the peers they go to for school help, personal help, and hanging out, as well as their perceptions of similarity to their student body as a whole, were included in this variable. The descriptive statistics for the Perceived similarity composite variable (M = 3.51 and SD = 0.85) indicated that the majority of students felt that just over half of their peers at school were similar to them ethnically and linguistically.

*Social Support at School.* In creating the five variables for perceived social support (Adult support for school help, Adult support for personal help, Peer support for school help, Peer support for personal help, Peer support for 'hanging out'), participants were asked, in open-ended manner, to report the number of people they turn to for different kinds of social support. For example, we asked: How many adults at school are you comfortable going to for personal help? (for example, when you need someone to talk to when you are mad, sad, or stressed). Due to several outliers, the data were recoded, such that high numbers were collapsed into the highest number before a natural break in the distribution. For example, in the case of the Adult support for school help variable, numbers 0–10 were counted as separate categories, and the final category, 11, included anyone who reported 11 individuals or more.

Descriptive analyses demonstrate that students reported that they would go to a median of 4 adults for school help (mean = 4.95, SD = 3.46), 1 adult for personal help (mean = 1.91, SD = 2.00), 9 peers for school help (mean = 7.98, SD = 4.56), 4 peers for personal help (mean = 5.02, SD = 4.13), and 11 peers for hanging out (mean = 9.33, SD = 4.25).

*Sense of School Belonging.* The Psychological Sense of School Membership scale (PSSM; Goodenow [1993]) was the outcome measure, and was used to determine adolescents' sense of school belonging. This scale was developed and validated with multi-ethnic, suburban and rural, middle and junior high school students [Goodenow, 1993]. The 18-item self-report PSSM uses a 5-point Likert scale, ranging from (1) 'not at all true' to (5) 'completely true'. The internal consistency score of 0.89 was obtained, which is comparable to that of other studies [Goodenow, 1993]. A mean composite School belonging variable was calculated. For the overall sample, participants, on average, felt that they 'somewhat' to 'mostly' belonged at their school (mean = 3.76, SD = 0.63).

*Data Analysis*

Hierarchical regressions were used to answer the research questions. The dependent variable was School belonging, and the independent variables were added as follows: In block 1 of the model, Gender, Grade, and Lone parenting (a proxy for SES) variables were added as covariates. To answer research question 1, the Racial/ethnic background dummy variables were then added in block 2, followed by the Generational status and Years in Canada variables entered in block 3. To answer Research question 2, Perceived similarity and School diversity were added in block 4 and the five social support variables were entered in block 5. Research question 3 involved a moderator analysis between time in Canada and social support variables. To analyze this, in block 6, all types of social support were moderated by Generation status. Although this final model involves the addition of several variables, using the formula provided by Tabachnick and Fidell [2001], it was determined that with 733 participants we had ample sample size and power to fit this model. In addition, in accordance with Aiken & West [1991], before entering the interaction terms, all variables from the previous model were first standardized in order avoid multicollinearity issues.

**Results**

Research question 1: How does length of time in Canada, generation status, and racial/ethnic background impact students' sense of school belonging?

To answer research question 1, the 'length of time in Canada', variables were entered into the model in block 3. Results indicated that after controlling for gender, age, ethnicity, and lone parent status, Generational status significantly predicted School belonging while Years in Canada did not. More specifically, Generational status was negatively associated with School belonging such that older generation students reported lower levels of school belonging. This significance held when the social context variables, Perceived similarity, and School diversity were entered (in block 4), but not when the social support variables were added in block 5 (see table 1).

Research question 2: In what ways does school social context and perceived social support impact School belonging?

To answer this research question, in block 4, the variables Perceived similarity and School diversity were entered into the model, and then in block 5 the five social support variables were entered. Perceived similarity significantly predicted School belonging such that feeling more similar, both ethnically and linguistically to one's peers was positively associated with School belonging.

It should be noted that the $R^2$ change value for Block 4 was modest but significant (see table 1, block 4) and Perceived similarity maintained its significant contribution in the final model (see table 1, block 5).

In block 5, the five types of social support variables were added. As can be seen from table 2, Adult support for school help and for personal help, and Peer support for 'hanging out' were positively associated with School belonging. These findings suggest that the more adult support for school help and personal help that participants perceived, the higher School belonging scores they reported. Similarly, the more peers that participants perceived they could hang out with, the higher School belonging scores they had.

Research question 3: Is the relationship between school social support and school belonging moderated by generation status?

To answer this research question, the interaction terms between each of the social support variables and Generational status were entered in block 6 (see table 2). As noted above, all of the previously entered variables were standardized before entering the interaction terms. Significant interactions were found between Adult support for school help and Generational status, as well as between Peer support for personal help and Generational status, all of which were significantly associated with School belonging (see table 2, block 6). After splitting Adult support for school help and Peer support for personal help into three groups (low, medium and high levels of support), the interactions were plotted for further analysis using Aiken & West's [1991] recommendations. As can be seen in figure 1, participants of each Generational status had a positive relationship between Adult support for school help and School belonging. That is, the more Adult support for school help they reported, the higher they scored on the School belonging scale. However, the difference lies in the slopes of the lines. Adolescents who had newly immigrated (1.5 generation Canadians) displayed a

**Table 1.** A hierarchical regression model summary representing sense of school belonging as predicted by social context variables at school (n = 733)

| Variables | Block 2[a] B | SE B | β | Block 3[a] B | SE B | β | Block 4[a] B | SE B | β | Block 5[a] B | SE B | β | $R^2$ | $\Delta R^2$ |
|---|---|---|---|---|---|---|---|---|---|---|---|---|---|---|
| Grade | −0.03 | 0.03 | −0.05 | −0.05 | 0.03 | −0.07 | −0.06 | 0.03 | −0.09 | −0.06 | 0.03 | −0.09* | 0.02 | 0.02* |
| Gender | −0.01 | 0.03 | −0.02 | −0.01 | 0.03 | −0.01 | −0.01 | 0.03 | −0.02 | 0.00 | 0.02 | 0.00 | | |
| Lone parent | −0.08 | 0.03 | −0.13** | −0.08 | 0.03 | −0.13** | −0.08 | 0.03 | −0.12** | −0.06 | 0.02 | −0.10** | | |
| European descent | 0.12 | 0.03 | 0.19*** | 0.16 | 0.03 | 0.26*** | 0.17 | 0.03 | 0.27*** | 0.11 | 0.03 | 0.17** | 0.05 | 0.03*** |
| Other descent | 0.08 | 0.03 | 0.13** | 0.10 | 0.03 | 0.16*** | 0.13 | 0.03 | 0.20*** | 0.10 | 0.03 | 0.16** | | |
| Years in Canada | | | | 0.04 | 0.03 | −0.06 | 0.04 | 0.03 | 0.06 | 0.02 | 0.03 | 0.03 | 0.05 | 0.00 |
| Generation status | | | | −0.08 | 0.04 | −0.12* | −0.10 | 0.04 | −0.16** | −0.07 | 0.04 | −0.10 | | |
| Perceived similarity | | | | | | | 0.08 | 0.03 | 0.12** | 0.07 | 0.03 | 0.11** | 0.06 | 0.01* |
| Adult school help | | | | | | | | | | 0.10 | 0.03 | 0.15** | 0.21 | 0.15*** |
| Adult personal help | | | | | | | | | | 0.10 | 0.03 | 0.14** | | |
| Peer school help | | | | | | | | | | 0.04 | 0.03 | 0.05 | | |
| Peer personal help | | | | | | | | | | 0.10 | 0.03 | 0.08 | | |
| Peer hanging out | | | | | | | | | | 0.10 | 0.03 | 0.14** | | |

* $p < 0.05$, ** $p < 0.01$, *** $p < 0.000$.
[a] These variables are standardized.

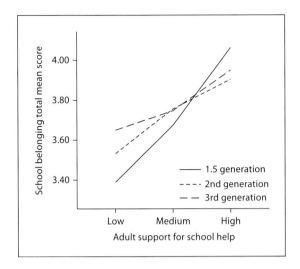

**Fig. 1.** The interaction between Generational status and Adult support for school help on sense of school belonging.

**Table 2.** Hierarchical regression moderator analysis where sense of school belonging is predicted by the interaction between Generation status and social support variables at school (n = 733)

| Variables | Block 5[a] | | | Block 6[a] | | | $R^2$ | $\Delta R^2$ |
|---|---|---|---|---|---|---|---|---|
| | B | SE B | β | B | SE B | β | | |
| Grade | −0.06 | 0.03 | −0.09* | −0.06 | 0.03 | −0.09* | 0.21 | 0.21*** |
| Gender | 0.00 | 0.02 | 0.00 | 0.00 | 0.02 | 0.00 | | |
| Lone parent | −0.06 | 0.02 | −0.10** | −0.06 | 0.02 | −0.10** | | |
| European descent | 0.11 | 0.03 | 0.17** | 0.11 | 0.03 | 0.17** | | |
| Other descent | 0.10 | 0.03 | 0.16** | 0.10 | 0.03 | 0.16** | | |
| Years in Canada | 0.02 | 0.03 | 0.03 | 0.02 | 0.03 | 0.03 | | |
| Generation status | −0.07 | 0.04 | −0.10 | −0.06 | 0.04 | −0.10 | | |
| Perceived similarity | 0.07 | 0.03 | 0.11** | 0.07 | 0.03 | 0.10** | | |
| Adult school help | 0.10 | 0.03 | 0.15** | 0.10 | 0.03 | 0.14** | | |
| Adult personal help | 0.10 | 0.03 | 0.14** | 0.10 | 0.03 | 0.15*** | | |
| Peer school help | 0.04 | 0.03 | 0.05 | 0.04 | 0.03 | 0.06 | | |
| Peer personal help | 0.10 | 0.03 | 0.08 | 0.05 | 0.03 | 0.07 | | |
| Peer hanging out | 0.10 | 0.03 | 0.14** | 0.10 | 0.23 | 0.15** | | |
| Adult school support × Gen | | | | −0.05 | 0.02 | −0.08* | 0.23 | 0.01* |
| Adult personal support × Gen | | | | 0.01 | 0.03 | 0.07 | | |
| Peer school support × Gen | | | | 0.00 | 0.02 | 0.01 | | |
| Peer personal support × Gen | | | | 0.06 | 0.03 | 0.10* | | |
| Peers for 'hanging out' × Gen | | | | −0.02 | 0.01 | −0.20 | | |

* $p < 0.05$, ** $p < 0.01$, *** $p < 0.001$.
[a] These variables are standardized.

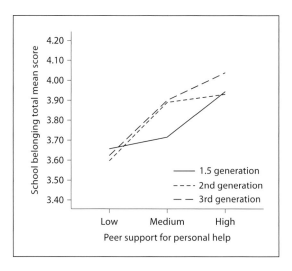

**Fig. 2.** The interaction between Generational status and Peer support for personal help on School belonging.

*Covariates*

As can be seen in table 1, block 1, Lone parenting was significantly associated with School belonging, such that adolescents who did not report having a lone parent tended to report higher scores on the School belonging scale (see table 1, block 5). It should be noted that Grade was not significantly associated with School belonging in block 1 (see table 1); however, in the final model, it significantly predicted School belonging with students in lower grades reporting higher feelings of school belonging. With the addition of Ethnicity variables in block 2, participants of European descent as well as Other descent reported higher scores on the School belonging scale compared to participants of Asian descent (the reference group), and this relationship held even after controlling for all of the other variables (see table 1, block 5).

stronger relationship between Adult support for school help and School belonging. More specifically, this group displayed the lowest scores on School belonging when Adult support for school help was low and the highest scores on School belonging when Adult support for school help was high. While the 2nd and 3rd generation groups had a less marked slope, the 3rd generation group showed slightly higher levels of school belonging than the 2nd generation group at both low and high levels of Adult support for school help.

Regarding Peer support for personal help, as can be seen in figure 2, at low levels of Peer support for personal help, the 1.5, 2nd, and 3rd generation groups displayed similar scores on School belonging. For medium levels of peer support for personal help at school, figure 2 illustrates a much sharper increase in School belonging in comparison to their 1.5 generation peers. In the presence of high levels of peer support for personal help, School belonging levels for 1.5 generation participants reaches that of their 2nd generation peers but does not match the higher levels School belonging found for the 3rd generation group.

**Discussion**

This study sought to determine the ways in which perceptions of school social context were associated with sense of school belonging for adolescents who are newcomers to Canada, in relation to those who are of earlier generations. The overall findings provided evidence in support of the immigrant paradox with more recent immigrant adolescents reporting higher levels of school belonging than those who were of earlier immigrant generations. To add complexity however, it was found that adolescents who were newer to Canada reported different levels of social support, and that they were impacted by this social support differently than those who were of earlier generations. In addition, it was found that certain aspects of students' perceived school social context affected their sense of school belonging more than other aspects. The specific findings are described below.

*School Belonging*

Generational status was significantly associated with participants' sense of school belonging, with newer generation Canadians reporting higher levels of School belonging. As noted above, this finding supports the immigrant paradox and rejects the notion of an assimilationist model of belonging, which assumes that the longer a person spends in a country, the better off they are [Harker, 2001]. Growing evidence in the Canadian context is finding that adolescents who are new to Canada are just as likely, or in some cases, more likely to succeed academically when compared with their peers who did not immigrate [Beiser, Hou, Hyman & Tousignant, 1998; McAndrew et al., 2009]. The current study suggests that the same pattern for academic success holds for adolescents who are new to Canada in terms of their levels of perceived school belonging.

Although much empirical work needs to be done to locate the specific reasons for the immigrant paradox, a few researchers have put forth their suggestions [Garcia Coll and Marks, in press]. One possible explanation comes from work suggesting that people who immigrate tend to create a strong familial network in response to the transition [Tseng, 2004]. The idea being that these individuals then receive the positive benefits typically associated with strong family ties. An extension of this is that children and adolescents in immigrant families tend to feel a strong sense of family obligation. This may translate into a strong motivation to succeed in their new school [Fuligni, Alvarez, Bachman & Ruble, 2005], and by extension, a person who is more engaged in a school is more likely to feel a sense of school belonging [Osterman, 2000]. Other research has also suggested that it is the potential for opportunity that a new country brings that facilitates optimism and success. Specifically, these researchers argue that people who immigrate are a self-selected group of individuals who are motivated to give their children a brighter future [Leventhal, Xue & Brooks-Gunn, 2006].

With the trend towards globalization, it is important to explain these findings through a more contextualized lens. There is a strong possibility that immigrant adolescents are already part of a new global generation that is comfortable with North American ideals and culture, by way of television, the Internet and other media, before arriving to the country. Because of this ability to begin the transition process prior to arriving, their already developed cultural competencies may allow them to transition with an ease that would not have been possible a decade ago. Furthermore, adolescents who immigrate are likely arriving in a country that is culturally more similar to their native country than it would have been in the past. Rising rates of immigration mean adolescents who immigrate may arrive to find many ethnically similar peers at their school and in their larger communities. Their immigration is part of a collective or group process that might be part of a long migratory history for that particular or similar ethnic groups. For many young immigrants, these ethnic enclaves can be helpful for newcomers in their process of adaptation to a new country as they can provide both social capital and access to critical resources [Portes & Zhou, 1993]. Irrespective of country of origin, new Canadians may be accepted by their peers who have undergone a similar immigration experience which may help to ease the transition process. All of the aforementioned theories may be at play in this study; however, only further research can truly unpack these hypotheses.

In considering the influence of both Racial/ethnic background and Generational status on adolescents' sense of school belonging, it is noteworthy that Generational status predicted students' School belonging over and above the effects of Ethnicity. In previous work, Generational status and minority status are factors that are often confounded in the literature [Quintana et al., 2006]. The current study provides evidence that these variables function differently and should therefore be considered as separate constructs. For example, being of Asian descent was associated with lower feelings of School belonging, while being new to Canada was associated with higher feelings of School belonging. This research indicates that there is something inherent in being new to a country, or the immigration experience, that is not explained by belonging to a certain ethnic group. The implications of generalizations across generations are many, providing a cautionary note for encompassing social categories that obscure immigration processes, i.e. Asian students.

Regarding the findings that were related to racial/ethnic background, participants of Asian descent, without taking into account generation status, reported significantly lower feelings of School belonging than their counterparts of any other descent (European or Other), even after controlling for gender, grade, and SES. This is despite the fact that students of Asian descent represented the largest proportion of participants and the largest proportion of students in the majority of the schools sampled (45.7%), and that students of East Asian descent, particularly from China, have a record across Canada and the US of excelling in their studies [Fuligni, 1998; McAndrew et al., 2009; Suarez-Orozco, Rhodes & Milburn, 2009]. Importantly, this academic success does not always translate to an overall positive school experience. In the context of the US, there is evidence to indicate that Asian students face higher levels of ethnic and racially based peer discrimination in comparison to their peers from other minority groups [Rosenbloom & Way, 2004]. They also report less comfort with racial features, and with peers that are not ethnically similar [Garcia Coll and Marks, 2009]. One of the factors that have been found to motivate their discrimination is their perceived higher levels of academic achievement, based on the 'model minority' stereotype [Qin, Way & Rana, 2008]. Further attention is warranted to undercover the extent to which lower sense of school belonging reported by students of Asian descent could be related to peer discrimination and harassment at school.

*The Impact of School Social Context*
As expected, Perceived similarity was positively related to students' sense of school belonging.

These findings are consistent with previous work that suggests adolescents are particularly sensitive to similarity [Bernt, 1981; Phan, 2003; Quillian & Campbell, 2003]. This may impact belonging for a few reasons: The importance of peer social relationships is characteristic of the developmental period of adolescence [Anderman, 2003], and attention to social similarity, such as ethnicity and language fluency, is thought to be heightened at this stage [Bellmore et al., 2007; Bernt, 1981; Tsai, 2006]. In fact, Benner & Graham [2007] found that ethnic incongruence was associated with lower feelings of school belonging. Additionally, research in the Canadian context has found evidence to indicate that adolescents who are new to Canada gained security and identity from networking with students who were culturally and linguistically similar to them [Hébert, 2005]. The findings here would suggest that students in schools in which they feel different from their peers may be at risk of feeling as if they do not belong. Knowing that same ethnicity and language peers provide social capital and critical resources related to academics and social customs [Portes & Rumbaut, 2001], a preliminary step would be to ensure that schools are prepared to provide these resources to newcomers. Most importantly, school leaders need to find ways of promoting a school culture in which difference is not only tolerated but becomes a source of pride.

Adult support for personal help was positively correlated with School belonging for the sample as a whole. This is not surprising in light of the large body of evidence citing teachers and other adults at school as unequivocally influential in students' perceptions of belonging at school [Furman & Buhrmester, 1992; for a review see Osterman, 2000]. This finding emphasizes the overall importance of adults at school and furthermore, their role in helping students when they are 'mad, sad, or stressed', as we defined Personal help in our study.

The interaction effect, showing that adolescents who were 1.5 generation Canadian (born outside of Canada) had a stronger relationship between adult support (for school help) and school belonging, is consistent with work done by Vedder, Boekart & Seegers [2005], who found that adolescents who immigrated placed a larger emphasis on teacher support than their non-immigrant counterparts. Interestingly, adolescents who immigrate have been found to rely on teacher support at school even more so than peer support for help [Morrison, Laughlin, San Miguel, Smith & Widaman, 1997]. The role of the teacher may be a reflection of traditional views of teachers in the country of origin, which are hypothesized to be transmitted from older generations [Garcia Coll and Marks, 2009]. Nevertheless, the eminent role of the teacher in students' sense of belonging at school, particularly for those who are new, reveals the importance of ensuring that they have access to this kind of support.

With respect to peer support, the amount of peers needed at school for personal help was moderated by their generation status. What figure 2 illustrates is that in the presence of medium levels of peer support for personal help at school, the 2nd and 3rd generation group seemed to gain more ground than the 1.5 generation group. Meaning, medium levels of peer support may not be sufficient for 1.5 generation adolescents to benefit from peer support for personal help at school. Indeed, social support is generally found to be positively correlated with psychological well-being of newcomers [Ward & Searle, 1991], and this also fits with school belonging research that suggests peer relationships are key to developing a sense of school belonging [Ryan, 2001]. The current study findings are most certainly in line with these findings, with the added insight that newcomers can feel a high sense of belonging at school but they may need more peer support and more specifically, more peer support for personal help (i.e. for when they are feeling mad, sad, or stressed).

It is interesting to note that, in contrast to Peer support for personal help, Peer support for school help was not found to significantly impact School belonging. This is consistent with research that shows that adolescents who immigrate rely on teacher support at school even more so than peer support for help [Morrison, Laughlin, San Miguel, Smith & Widaman, 1997]. Still, peers have been found to play an important role in the academic achievement of those who immigrate [Fuligni, 1997]. It may be the case that school help by peers is sourced from places other than school, for example, in the community or from family members [Faircloth & Hamm, 2005]. Another possibility is that while peer support for school help may be critical to academic outcomes, it may not be a necessary component to feeling a sense of belonging at school.

*Limitations*
This work is very timely given the increase of immigrants to Canada; however, it does not come without some limitations. A cultural limitation of this study was that the smaller racial/ethnic background groupings were not analyzed as individual groups because of their small numbers. As a result, these ethnic groups were compiled to create an Other ethnicity category. In the future, a larger, more heterogeneous sample will enable distinctions among various ethnicities. Smaller groups, such as students from Middle Eastern and African/Caribbean descent, are underrepresented not only in the schools but also in our sample. Unfortunately, it is likely that these students are the ones who feel the least similar to their peers and, as such, may be most vulnerable to feeling as though they do not belong at school. It is worth noting that this trend was evident in the current data set, albeit insignificant with such small sample sizes. The current study was based on adolescent self-reports. Considering the social nature of the study, the use of multiple informants would certainly strengthen the findings. In addition to this, a wider age range of participants would provide an enhanced ability to interpret across a wider span of development.

## Future Directions and Conclusion

The trends in the current study, as well as in extant research, suggest that the gains made by the first generation may be lost by the second generation [for example, Harker, 2001]. Future research that focuses specifically on needs of further generations of newcomers (i.e. 2nd and 3rd generation Canadians) and the factors that lead to their documented declines in achievement and perhaps social-emotional functioning at school is required. In tangent with this, and in light of the findings of the current study and past research which suggest immigration status is associated with positive academic outcomes and perhaps even a developmental advantage, future research needs to focus on disentangling the specific protective and resiliency factors that seem to be associated with this emerging pattern.

We would like to highlight three main considerations, each of which is important to researchers, practitioners, and policy-makers alike. First, the current study showed that it is not only peers who define adolescents' school belonging experience, but adults at school as well. This is especially marked if adolescents are newer to Canada. Second, it is imperative to note that although most students in the current study do seem to feel a sense of school belonging, there are certainly adolescents who do not. It is essential to pay attention to these cases and consider why it is that these individuals are not having their needs met. Finally, we cannot assume that all adolescents require the same things from their school. Social contextual factors at school are evidently a substantial part of all adolescents' experience of school belonging. If we are to create exceptional schools that cater to the needs of individual students, then, based on the current findings, it is essential to bear in mind that some adolescents, such as those who are newer to Canada, have different social needs, and, therefore, require different types and amounts of support.

## References

Aiken, L.S., & West, S.G. (1991). *Multiple regression: Testing and interpreting interactions.* London: Sage Publications.

Alegria, M., Sribney, W., Woo, M., Torres, M., & Guarnaccia, P. (2007). Looking beyond nativity: The relation of age of immigration, length of residence, and birth cohorts to the risk of onset of psychiatric disorders for Latinos. *Research in Human Development, 4,* 19–47.

Anderman, L.H. (2003). Academic and social perceptions as predictors of change in middle school students' sense of belonging. *The Journal of Experimental Education, 72,* 5–22.

Anderman, L.H., & Freeman, T. (2004). Students' sense of belonging in school. In M.L. Maehr & P.R. Pintrich (Eds.), *Advances in motivation and achievement. Vol. 13. Motivating students, improving schools: The legacy of Carol Midgley* (pp. 27–63). Oxford: Elsevier.

Bailey, B.H. (2001). Dominican-American ethnic/racial identities and United States social categories. *International Migration Review, 35,* 677–708.

Baumeister, R.F., & Leary, M.R. (1995). The need to belong: Desire for interpersonal attachments as a fundamental human motivation. *Psychological Bulletin, 117,* 497–529.

Beiser, M., Hou, F., Hyman, I., & Tousignant, M. (1998). Growing Up Canadian: A study of immigrant children. Applied Resource Branch, Strategic Policy: Human Resources Development Canada.

Beiser, M., Hou, F., Hyman, I., & Tousignant, M. (2002). Poverty, family process, and the mental health of immigrant children in Canada. *American Journal of Public Health, 92,* 220–227.

Bellmore, A.D., Nishina, A., Witkow, M.R., Graham, S., & Juvoven, J. (2007). The influence of classroom ethnic composition on same- and other-ethnicity peer nominations in middle school. *Social Development, 16,* 720–740.

Benner, A.D., & Graham, S. (2007). Navigating the transition to multi-ethnic urban high schools: Changing ethnic congruence and adolescents' school-related affect. *Journal of Research on Adolescence, 17,* 207–220.

Bernt, T.J. (1981). Age changes and changes over time in prosocial intentions and behavior between friends. *Developmental Psychology, 17,* 408–416.

Berry, J.W., Westin, C., Virta, E., Vedder, P., Rooney, R., & Sang, D. (2006). Design of the study: Selecting societies of settlement and immigrant groups. In J.W. Berry, J.S. Phinney, D.L. Sam & P. Vedder (Eds.), *Immigrant youth in cultural transition: Acculturation, identity, and adaptation across national contexts* (pp. 15–45). Mahwah: Lawrence Erlbaum, Associates.

Certo, J.L., Cauley, K.M., & Chafin, C. (2003). Students' perspectives on their high school experience. *Adolescence, 38,* 705–724.

Chen, X. (2001). Group social functioning and individual socioemotional and school adjustment in Chinese children. *Merrill-Palmer Quarterly, 47*, 264–299.

Chen, J., Ng, E., & Wilkins, R. (1996). The health of Canada's immigrants in 1994–95. *Health Reports, 7*, 33–45.

Chiu, M.L., Feldman, S.S., & Rosenthal, D.A. (1992). The influence of immigration on parental behavior and adolescent distress in Chinese families residing in two western nations. *Journal of Research on Adolescence, 2*, 205–239.

Citizenship and Immigration Canada (2006). Final report: G8 experts roundtable on diversity and integration. The metropolis secretariat, Citizenship and Immigration Canada. Retrived on Sept. 31, 2007, from http://canada.metropolis.net/publications/G8_Report_Eng.pdf.

Coleman, J. (1961). *The adolescent society*. Glencoe, New York.

Crosnoe, R. (2006). Health and the education of children from racial/ethnic minority and immigrant families. *Journal of Health and Behavior, 47*, 77–93.

Eccles, J., & Midgley, C. (1989). Stage/environment fit: Developmentally appropriate classrooms for early adolescents. In R. Ames & C. Ames (Eds.), *Research on motivation in education. Vol. 3* (pp. 139–186). New York: Academic Press.

Elias, M.J. (2006). The connection between academic and social-emotional learning. In M.J. Elias & H. Arnold (Eds.), *The educator's guide to emotional intelligence and academic achievement.* Thousand Oaks: Corwin Press.

Faircloth, B.S., & Hamm, J.V. (2005). Sense of belonging among high school students representing 4 ethnic groups. *Journal of Youth and Adolescence, 34*, 293–309.

Fuligni, A. (1998). The adjustment of children from immigrant families. *Current Directions in Psychological Science, 7*, 99–103.

Fuligni, A.J. (1997). The academic achievement of adolescents from immigrant families: The roles of family background, attitudes, and behavior. *Child Development, 68*, 351–363.

Fuligni, A.J., Alvarez, J., Bachman, M., & Ruble, D.N. (2005). Family obligation and the academic motivations of young children from immigrant families. In C.R. Cooper, C. Garcia Coll, T. Bartko, H. Davis & C. Chatman (Eds.), *Hills of gold: Rethinking diversity and contexts as resources for children's developmental pathways.* Mahwah, NJ: Lawrence Erlbaum Associates.

Furman, W., & Buhrmester, D. (1992). Age and sex differences in perceptions of networks of personal relationships. *Child Development, 63*, 103–115.

Garcia Coll, C., Lamberty, G., Jenkins, G., McAdoo, H.P., Crnic, K., Wasik, B.H., et al. (1996). An integrative model for the study of developmental competencies in minority children. *Child Development, 67*, 1891–1914.

Garcia Coll, C., & Marks, A.K. (eds). The immigrant paradox: is becoming American a developmental risk? American Psychological Association, Washington, D.C. (in press).

Garcia Coll, C., & Marks, A.K. (2009). Immigrant Stories: Ethnicity and academics in middle childhood. New York: Oxford University Press.

Goodenow, C. (1993). The psychological sense of school membership among adolescents: Scale development and educational correlates. *Psychology in the Schools, 30*, 79–90.

Graham, J.A., & Cohen, R. (1997). Race and sex as factors in children's sociometric ratings and friendship choices. *Social Development, 6*, 355–372.

Han, W.-J. (2008). The academic trajectories of children of immigrants and their school environments. *Developmental Psychology, 44*, 1572–1590.

Harker, K. (2001). Immigrant generation, assimilation, and adolescent psychological well-being. *Social Forces, 79*, 969–1004.

Hébert, Y. (2005). Transculturalism among Canadian youth focus on strategic competence and social capital. In D. Hoerder, Y. Hebert, & I. Schmitt (Eds.), *Negotiating transcultural lives: Belongings and social capital among youth in comparative perspective* (pp. 103–128). Toronto: University of Toronto Press.

Hernandez, D.J. (2004). Demographic change and the life circumstances of immigrant families. *Future of Children, 14*, 17–47.

Hernandez, M.Y. (2009). Psychological theories of immigration. *Journal of Human Behavior in the Social Environment, 19*, 713–729.

Hough, R.L., Hazen, A.L., Soriano, F.I., Wood, P., McCabe, K., & Yeh, M. (2002). Mental health care for Latinos: Mental health services for Latino adolescents with psychiatric disorders. *Psychiatric Services, 53*, 1556–1562.

Hymel, S., Schonert-Reichl, K., & Miller, L. (2007). Reading, 'riting, 'rithmetic and relationships: Considering the social side of education. *Exceptionality Education Canada, 16*, 149–192.

Kao, G. (1999). Psychological well-being and educational achievement among immigrant youth. In D. J. Hernandez (Ed.), *Children of immigrants: Health, adjustment, and public assistance.* Washington: National Academy Press.

Kao, G., & Tienda, M. (1995). Optimism and achievement: The educational performance of immigrant youth. *Social Science Quarterly, 76*, 1–19.

Kiang, L., & Fuligni, A. (2009). Ethnic identity in context: Variations in ethnic exploration and belonging with parent, same-ethnic, and different-ethnic peer relationships. *Journal of Youth and Adolescence, 38*, 732–743.

Ladd, G.W. (1990). Having friends, keeping friends, making friends, and being liked by peers in the classroom: Predictors of children's early school adjustment? *Child Development, 61*, 1081–1100.

Leventhal, T., Xue, Y., & Brooks-Gunn, J. (2006). Immigrant differences in school-age children's verbal trajectories: A look at four racial/ethnic groups. Child Development, 77, 1359–1374.

Maehr, M.L., & Midgley, C. (1996). Transforming school cultures. Boulder, CO: Westview Press.

McAndrew, M., Ait-Said, R., Ledent, J., Murdoch, J., Anisef, P., Brown, R., Sweet, R., Walters, D., Aman, C., & Garnett, B. (2009). *Educational pathways of youth of immigrant origin: Comparing Montreal, Toronto, and Vancouver.* Ottawa: Canadian Council on Learning.

McDonald, J.T., & Kennedy, S. (2004). Insights into the 'healthy immigrant effect': health status and health service use of immigrants to Canada. *Social Science & Medicine, 59*, 1613–1627.

McDougall, P., Hymel, S., Vaillancourt, T., & Mercer, L. (2001). The consequences of childhood peer rejection. In M. Leary (Ed.), *Interpersonal rejection* (pp. 213–247). New York: Oxford University Press.

Morrison, G.M., Laughlin, J., San Miguel, S., Smith, D.C., & Widamin, K. (1997). Sources of support for school-related issues: Choices of Hispanic adolescents varying in migrant status. *Journal of Youth and Adolescence, 26*, 233–252.

National Research Council. (2007). *Understanding interventions that encourage minorities to pursue research careers: Summary of a workshop*. Retrieved October 10, 2008, from http://dels.nas.edu/dels/rpt_briefs/MORE_workshop_final.pdf.

Onyekwuluje, A.B. (1998). Multiculturalism, diversity, and the impact parents and schools have on societal race relations. *The School Community Journal, 8*, 55–71.

Osterman, K.F. (2000). Students' need for belonging in the school community. *Review of Educational Research, 70*, 323–367.

Perez, C. (2002). Health status and health behaviour among immigrants. *Health Reports (suppl), Vol. 13*. Statistics Canada, Catalogue 82–003.

Phan, T. (2003). Life in school: Narratives of resiliency among Vietnamese Canadian youths. *Adolescence, 38*, 555–566.

Piaget, J. (1932). *The moral judgment of the child*. Glencoe, IL: Free Press.

Portes, A. (2000). The two meanings of social capital. *Sociological Forum, 15*, 1–12.

Portes, A., & Rumbaut, R. (2001). *Legacies: The story of the immigrant second generation*. Berkeley: University of California Press.

Portes, A., & Zhou, M. (1993). The new second generation: Segmented assimilation and its variants among post-1965 immigrant youth. *Annals of the American Academy of Political and Social Science, 530*, 74–98.

Qin, D.B., Way, N., & Rana, M. (2008). The 'model minority' and their discontent: Examining peer discrimination and harassment of Chinese American immigrant youth. In H. Yoshikawa & N. Way (Eds.), Beyond the family: Contexts of immigrant children's development. *New Directions for Child and Adolescent Development, 121*, 27–42.

Quillan, L., & Campbell, M.E. (2003). Beyond black and white: The present and future of multiracial friendship segregation. *American Sociological Review, 68*, 540–556.

Quintana, S.M., Aboud, F.E., Chao, R.K., Contreras-Grau, J., Cross Jr., W.E., Hudley, C., et al., (2006). Race, ethnicity, and culture in child development: Contemporary research and future directions. *Child Development, 77*, 1129–1141.

Raffo, C., & Reeves, M. (2000). Youth transitions and social exclusion: Developments in social capital theory. *Journal of Youth Studies, 3*, 147–166.

Rogoff, B. (1990). *Apprenticeship in thinking*. New York: Oxford University Press.

Rosenbloom, S.R., & Way, N. (2004). Experiences of discrimination among African American, Asian American, and Latino adolescents in an urban high school. *Youth & Society, 35*, 420–451.

Rotheram, M.J., & Phinney, J. (1987). Introduction: Definitions and perspectives in the study of children's ethnic socialization. In J. Phinney & M.J. Rotheram (Eds.), *Children's ethnic socialization: Pluralism and development* (pp. 10–28). Beverley Hills: Sage.

Rubin, K.H., Bukowski, W., & Parker, J.G. (1998). Peer interactions, relationships, and groups. In N. Eisenberg (Ed.), *Handbook of child psychology. Vol. 3: Social, emotional, and personality development* (pp. 619–700). New York: Wiley.

Rumbaut, R.G. (2008). Divergent destinies: Acculturation, social mobility, and adult transitions among Latin American and Asian immigrants. Invited address at the meeting of the Society for Research on Adolescence, Chicago, USA.

Ryan, R.M. (1995). Psychological needs and the facilitation of integrative processes. *Journal of Personality, 63*, 397–427.

Ryan, A.M. (2001). The peer group as a context for the development of young adolescent motivation and achievement. *Child Development, 72*, 1135–1150.

Sonderegger, R., Barrett, P.M., & Creed, P.A. (2004). Models of cultural adjustment for child and adolescent migrants to Australia: Internal process and situational factors. *Journal of Child and Family Studies, 13*, 357–371.

Suarez-Orozco, C., & Carhill, A. (2008). Afterword: New directions in research with immigrant families and their children. In H. Yoshikawa & N. Way (Eds.), Beyond the family: Contexts of immigrant children's development. *New Directions for Child and Adolescent Development, 121*, 87–104.

Suarez-Orozco, C., Gaytan, F.X., Bang, H.J., Pakes, J., O'Connor, E., & Rhodes, J. (2010). Academic trajectories of newcomer immigrant youth. *Developmental Psychology, 46*, 602–618.

Suarez-Orozco, C., Qin-Hilliard, D.B. (2004). The cultural psychology of academic engagement: Immigrant boys' experiences in U.S. schools. In N. Way & J. Chu (Eds.), *Adolescent boys: Exploring diverse cultures of boyhood*. New York: New York University Press.

Suarez-Orozco, C., Rhodes, J., & Milburn, M. (2009). Unravelling the immigrant paradox: Academic engagement and disengagement among recently arrived immigrant youth. *Youth & Society, 41*, 151–185.

Suarez-Orozco, C., & Suarez-Orozco, M. (2001). *Children of immigration*. Cambridge, MA: Harvard University Press.

Sullivan, H.S. (1953). *The interpersonal theory of psychiatry*. New York: Norton.

Tabachnick, B.G., & Fidell, L.S. (2001). *Using multivariate statistics* (4th ed.). Chicago: Allyn and Bacon.

Takeuchi, D.T., Hong, S., Gile, K., & Alegria, M. (2007). Developmental contexts and mental disorders among Asian Americans. *Research in Human Development, 4*, 49–69.

Tatum, B.D. (1999). *Why are all the Black kids sitting together in the cafeteria? and other conversations about race*. New York: Basic Books.

Tsai, H-S. (2006). Xenophobia, ethnic community, and immigrant youths' friendship network formation. *Adolescence, 41*, 285–298.

Tseng V. (2004). Family interdependence and academic adjustment in college: Youth from immigrant and U.S.-born families. *Child Development, 75*, 966–983.

Vedder, P., Boekarts, M., & Seegers, G. (2005). Perceived social support and well-being in school: The role of students' ethnicity. *Journal of Youth and Adolescence, 34*, 269–278.

Ward, C., & Searle, W. (1991). The impact of value discrepancies and cultural identity on psychological and sociocultural adjustment of sojourners. International *Journal of Intercultural Relations, 15*, 209–225.

Watson, M., Battistich, V., & Solomon, D. (1997). Enhancing students' social and ethnical development in school: An intervention program and its effects. *International Journal of Educational Research, 27*, 571–586.

Wenz-Gross, M., Siperstein, G.M., Untch, A.S., & Widaman, K.F. (1997). Stress, social support, and the adjustment of adolescents in middle school. *Journal of Early Adolescence, 17,* 129–151.

Yoshikawa, H., & Way, N. (2008). From peers to policy: How broader social contexts influence the adaptation of children and youth in immigrant families. In H. Yoshikawa & N. Way (Eds.), *Beyond the family: Contexts of immigrant children's development. New Directions for Child and Adolescent Development, 121,* 1–8.

Zins, J.E., Bloodworth, M.R., Weissberg, R.P., & Walberg, H.J. (2004). The scientific base linking social and emotional learning to school success. In J.E. Zins, R.P. Weissberg, M.C. Wang, H.J. Walberg (Eds.), *Building academic success on social and emotional learning: What does the research say?* New York: Teachers College Press.

Monique Gagné
Department of Education and Couns. Psych., and Spec. Education, University of British Columbia
Vancouver, BC V6T1Z4 (Canada)
E-Mail mgagne@interchange.ubc.ca

# Are Immigrant Children in Italy Better Adjusted than Mainstream Italian Children?

Radosveta Dimitrova · Athanasios Chasiotis

Tilburg University, Tilburg, The Netherlands

## Abstract

The purpose of this study was to examine the association of immigrant status with psychosocial adjustment in Albanian and Serbian immigrants compared to Slovene and Italian mainstream children by addressing the research question: How is psychosocial adjustment in immigrant children in Italy associated with their ethnic background and gender? Four groups of 7- to 12-year-old pupils of first-generation Albanian (n = 152) and Serbian immigrants (n = 124), and Italian (n = 300) and Slovene (n = 64) mainstream children were studied. Self- and teacher reports were collected regarding children's social (emotional instability, prosocial and aggressive behavior) and psychological (depressive symptoms) adjustment. Results revealed that in spite of lower socioeconomic status, immigrant children, but not their teachers, reported lower levels of emotional instability and aggression. Gender comparisons showed that boys scored higher on emotional instability, aggression, and lower on prosocial behavior than girls. Overall, results of children's self-reports suggest that Albanian and Serbian children feel positively about their social relationships in the country of settlement; however, these behavioral patterns go largely undetected by teachers. Findings and their implications for possible social desirability effects on the observed differences are discussed.

Copyright © 2012 S. Karger AG, Basel

Research on adaptation of immigrants is growing, especially among adolescents. However, there is little on immigrants into Italy and little on prepubertal immigrants. In addition, there is a conflict in the literature regarding whether immigrants adapt better or worse than their native counterparts. The aim of this study is to fill this gap by investigating social and psychological adjustment among Italian prepubertal immigrants.

Extensive research has identified divergent pathways in adjustment of immigrant children in their new culture. The *migration-morbidity* hypothesis and the *selective-migration hypothesis* are two potential explanations for these differential findings. The first hypothesis states that there is a strong relationship between migrant status and psychological morbidity, leading to psychosocial problems in immigrant populations [Klimidis, Stuart, Minas & Ata, 1994], whereas the second one contends that migration does not necessarily increase the risk for psychological or behavioral difficulties because of various protective factors such as positive family functioning, strong social networks and shared financial resources [Fichter, Xepapadakos, Quadflieg, Georgopoulou & Fthenakis, 2004].

Regarding the migration-morbidity hypothesis, numerous studies across various cultures have documented the prevalence of psychosocial adjustment difficulties in immigrant samples. There is evidence showing that children from different cultural backgrounds living in a variety of cultural settings show more psychological problems [Derluyn & Broekaert, 2007; Leavey et al., 2004; Stevens et al., 2003], delinquent and aggressive behavior [Janssen et al., 2004] and generally higher distress rates than those of their non-immigrant peers. Whereas much of the research examining the migration-morbidity hypothesis suggests that immigration and consequent acculturation experience are essentially stressful, recent evidence has challenged the notion of inexorable migration effects on an individual psychological functioning. Accordingly, despite higher risk factors of family poverty and neighborhood disadvantage, some immigrant youths relative to native youths have been reported to experience less emotional [Beiser, Hou, Hyman & Tousignant, 2002; Harker, 2001] and behavioral problems [Georgiades, Boyle & Duku, 2007; Strohmeier, Spiel & Gradinger, 2008]. Such 'healthy migrant effect' related to disadvantaged socioeconomic conditions of immigrant populations is often referred to as the *immigrant paradox*. Obviously, the counterintuitive nature makes such finding especially interesting, as positive health outcomes of immigrants do not correspond to their lower socioeconomic status (SES) or the stresses associated with being an immigrant.

What makes the latter findings more complex to interpret is the fact that data in the international literature concerning psychosocial adjustment outcomes of immigrant children are contradictory. Some authors report that immigrant groups surveyed in their countries do better than natives in both sociocultural adaptation [Sam, Vedder, Liebkind, Neto & Virta, 2008] and psychological adaptation [Slodnjak, Kos & Yule, 2002], whereas others report exactly the opposite [Derluyn & Broekaert, 2007; Janssen et al., 2004]. Additionally, research suggests that gender influences children's outcomes such that contrary to findings in the US in which girls show more depressive symptoms, immigrant boys show higher depressive symptoms [Holmberg & Hellberg, 2008] and higher behavioral problems compared to immigrant girls [Derluyn, Broekaert & Schuyten, 2008].

Research has also produced contradictory results due to different informants. For example, negative migration impact on children's adjustment has been found in parents and teachers' reports but not in self-reports. A study conducted by Stevens et al. [2003] in the Netherlands revealed that, compared to the Dutch group, Turkish and Moroccan immigrant children showed higher levels of internalizing and externalizing problems as reported by parents and teachers, respectively. In contrast, the immigrant children themselves reported fewer emotional and behavioral problems compared to native Dutch children. Other studies using teacher reports show mixed evidence, suggesting fewer psychological problems [Loo & Rapport, 1998] or no differences in problem behaviors between immigrant and native children [Crijnen, Bengi-Arslan & Verhulst, 2000].

Much less is known about immigrant youth in Italy, where the percentage of children from immigrant families is constantly increasing. Albanians and Serbians constitute major ethnic groups among Italian immigrants, especially in the North-Eastern region, representing 13 and 10% of the immigrant population, respectively [National Statistic Institute, 2010]. They also belong to the socially disadvantaged immigrants, negatively stereotyped by the dominant Italian majority, although they differ in their acculturation because Serbian immigration has a long-term history stemming from economic reasons and family reunifications, whereas the Albanian immigration is a more recent phenomenon linked to refugee displacement in the early 1990s [Mai & Schwandner-Sievers, 2003]. Additionally to these immigrant groups, we also considered children belonging to the Slovene ethnic community, representing a native-born bilingual group residing only in the Northeastern part of the country with a peculiar minority status compared to the local Italian population. We included this group because of its distinctive features of bicultural indigenous minority representing an integral part of the multiethnic composition of the local population. Slovenes are a bilingual minority linguistically similar but ethnically diverse from the Italian majority and at the same time, a native community compared to both Albanian and Serbian immigrants.

A further strength of this study regards the age of the participants. Most studies on adjustment outcomes of immigrant children have been carried out almost exclusively with adolescents [Fuligni, 1997; Portes & Rumbaut, 2001]. No study has yet examined the psychological and social adjustment of prepubertal children of immigrants from different cultural backgrounds in Italy. Middle childhood between ages 6 and 12 is a crucial period marked by developmental sensibility with important implications for the future [García Coll & Szalacha, 2004]. It is during this stage that children develop abilities in different domains and interactions with environments outside of their families. Children's self-perception within different contexts emerges in that period, influencing positive attitudes toward school and future aspirations, which can have a significant impact on their future as successful adults. If issues are identified earlier in life, preventive interventions could be implemented to ameliorate negative long-term outcomes.

Finally, a distinctive characteristic of the study regards the inclusion of an external validation of children's self-reports on adjustment. Therefore, obtaining supplementary information by sources other than the respondent's report contributes to the accuracy of comparative acculturation studies [Arends-Tóth & van de Vijver, 2006; van de Vijver, Hofer & Chasiotis, 2010]. Because self-reports are one of the most extensively used techniques as a source of psychological information, an important concern is to what extent children are capable to report their actual difficulties accurately. To address this concern we employed both self- and teacher reports on social adjustment of the immigrant and native children.

In conclusion, existing research indicates that the adaptation of immigrant populations is influenced by different sources of information, gender and ethnicity in a complex way. In addressing these issues, the present study attempts to bring together contextual and comparative aspects of multiple groups of minority children, which have not been considered in a single study before. Specifically, we compare the psychological and social adjustment of Albanian and Serbian immigrant school-aged children with their mainstream Slovenian and Italian peers, and explore how these outcomes are affected by gender and ethnic background.

## Context and Hypotheses

Italy with its native population of about 60 million has turned from a traditionally country of emigration to that of immigration, where foreigners represent 7% (4,330,000) of the total population [Caritas e Migrantes, 2009]. Additionally, the ethnic diversity within the country has increased very rapidly and particularly in the Northeastern region, which presents two characteristics attractive for migration. One is its geographic proximity to the Balkan States, which facilitates migratory movements from Eastern Europe (Albania and former Yugoslavia). Another concerns good local economic growth and better labor opportunities, contributing to a stable settlement for immigrant families in that area [Marra, 2002].

It is also of interest that Albanians and Serbians share common low status-relevant dimensions as minorities in the system of social hierarchy – they are the largest and most representative ethnicities associated with difficult socioeconomic circumstances, social exclusion and negative stereotyping by the dominant Italian majority [Mai & Schwandner-Sievers, 2003].

Still, both cultural background and contextual characteristics of these groups vary considerably in terms of migration history and social status. The Serbian community has a long-term migration movement to Northeastern Italy, which is supported by extensive social networks and a cohesive Serbian receiving community. Compared with the Albanian group in the area, therefore, Serbians have had the longest time to adapt to the Italian society, and at the same time they have been able to maintain their cultural heritage. In Northeastern Italy, there are Orthodox Serbian-language churches, local businesses, educational and community organizations available to serve the immigrant Serbian population [Marra, 2002].

Conversely, the settling of Albanians in Italy is a more recent phenomenon with the first migrations occurring in the early 1990s, following changes within the political system in their home country. Albanians are more vulnerable to pronounced negative stereotyping and discrimination than are Serbians [King & Mai, 2009] because of the greater prevalence of undocumented or refugees in their community and related labor inclusion challenges.

In contrast to Albanian and Serbian immigrant communities who emigrated from their home countries to Italy, Slovenes are a native population who remained on Italian territory after the delimitation of the border between Italy and former Yugoslavia in 1919. Slovenes are the dominant and the most numerous bilingual community in north-eastern region owning a particular minority status with the adoption of the Law on the Protection of Slovene Ethnic Minority in 2001. They have developed various political, economic and sociocultural networks – all factors which significantly contribute to their integration within the Italian majority context [Brezigar, 1999]. We include them because of distinctive characteristics of this bilingual and indigenous ethnic minority in the context in which the study was conducted.

This study aims to investigate the following research question: How is psychosocial adjustment in immigrant children in Italy associated with their ethnic background and gender? If the migration morbidity hypothesis is supported, immigrant children compared to mainstream children will show higher adjustment problems, whereas we expect lower adjustment problems in the immigrant rather than in the mainstream group if the selective migration hypothesis holds true. Furthermore, we expect that Serbian children will show higher adjustment levels compared to their Albanian peers and that boys will manifest more problems in psychosocial components than girls. Because of a less successful integration of the Albanian community in Italy, we assume that Albanian boys would show the highest levels of adjustment difficulties.

## Method

*Participants*

The total sample consisted of 640 children (7–12 years old, mean age: 9.10) of varied ethnicities: Albanian (n = 152), Serbian (n = 124), Italian (n = 300) and Slovene (n = 64; table 1). All participants were attending different elementary schools located in the Northeastern region of Italy, and all immigrant children had been living in Italy for one to up to 10 years. With the help of school personnel, immigrant children who potentially met the inclusion criteria (first-generation immigrants whose parents were both from the same country of origin, i.e. Albania and Serbia) were identified. Prior to data collection, teachers were asked about the average length of stay of the immigrant children, thereby including only those who were residing in Italy for at least one academic year. School registers containing occupation status of both parents were used to obtain information about the participants' family SES. The three categories of low, middle and high SES were based on the Italian National Statistic Institute for occupational classifications [Scarnera, 2001].

Analysis of variance revealed significant differences between the four cultural groups with respect to age of participants with the Italian being about 3 months younger than Albanian, Serbian and Slovene children, $F(3, 639) = 4.14$, $p < 0.001$. Because analyses testing age effects on adjustment outcome variables did not show

**Table 1.** Descriptive statistics of the sample by ethnic group

|  | Albanian | Serbian | Slovene | Italian | Total |
|---|---|---|---|---|---|
| Male/female | 65/87 | 59/65 | 32/32 | 125/175 | 281/359 |
| Age, years |  |  |  |  |  |
|   Range | 7–12 | 7–12 | 7–12 | 7–12 | 7–12 |
|   Mean (SD) | 9.34 (1.47) | 9.21 (1.50) | 9.27 (1.15) | 8.89 (1.37) | 9.10 (1.41) |
| SES |  |  |  |  |  |
|   Low | 105 (78%) | 81 (69%) | 17 (27%) | 80 (28%) | 283 (47%) |
|   Middle | 29 (21%) | 35 (30%) | 31 (48%) | 168 (60%) | 263 (44%) |
|   High | 1 (0.7%) | 1 (0.9%) | 16 (25%) | 34 (12%) | 52 (9%) |
| Length of residence |  |  |  |  |  |
|   1–5 years | 114 (83%) | 81 (71%) | – | – | 195 (78%) |
|   5–10 years | 23 (17%) | 33 (29%) | – | – | 56 (22%) |
| CSACIQ-SR |  |  |  |  |  |
|   Emotional instability |  |  |  |  |  |
|     Mean (SD) | 17.50 (4.05) | 17.37 (4.05) | 18.46 (4.05) | 19.23 (4.20) | 18.38 (4.20) |
|     Cronbach's alpha | 0.79 | 0.78 | 0.82 | 0.81 | 0.81 |
|   Prosocial behavior |  |  |  |  |  |
|     Mean (SD) | 20.19 (2.80) | 20.72 (2.53) | 20.73 (2.92) | 21.03 (2.51) | 20.74 (2.64) |
|     Cronbach's alpha | 0.70 | 0.65 | 0.75 | 0.66 | 0.69 |
|   Aggression |  |  |  |  |  |
|     Mean (SD) | 13.49 (3.49) | 12.79 (3.37) | 14.30 (3.47) | 14.36 (3.93) | 13.84 (3.79) |
|     Cronbach's alpha | 0.83 | 0.78 | 0.81 | 0.82 | 0.82 |
| CDI |  |  |  |  |  |
|   Depression |  |  |  |  |  |
|     Mean (SD) | 10.54 (5.03) | 9.94 (5.11) | 8.52 (6.40) | 9.14 (6.30) | 9.60 (5.84) |
|     Cronbach's alpha | 0.69 | 0.71 | 0.85 | 0.82 | 0.79 |
| CSACIQ-TR |  |  |  |  |  |
|   Emotional instability |  |  |  |  |  |
|     Mean (SD) | 17.21 (5.71) | 17.02 (5.07) | 18.41 (4.46) | 17.21 (5.71) | 17.27 (5.22) |
|     Cronbach's alpha | 0.69 | 0.80 | 0.79 | 0.80 | 0.92 |
|   Prosocial behavior |  |  |  |  |  |
|     Mean (SD) | 19.26 (2.67) | 19.00 (2.98) | 18.75 (3.14) | 19.77 (3.14) | 19.35 (2.94) |
|     Cronbach's alpha | 0.91 | 0.91 | 0.94 | 0.93 | 0.76 |
|   Aggression |  |  |  |  |  |
|     Mean (SD) | 11.18 (3.68) | 11.20 (3.47) | 12.57 (4.34) | 11.72 (4.27) | 11.62 (4.02) |
|     Cronbach's alpha | 0.88 | 0.85 | 0.94 | 0.80 | 0.85 |

statistically significant results, further analyses did not control for age. No culture-related differences emerged for the distribution of gender, $\chi^2$ (3, n = 640) = 2.33, p = 0.506 (see table 1). Finally, cultural groups differed with respect to family SES [$\chi^2$ (6, n = 598) = 143.56; p < 0.001], with Italian children having higher SES. All subsequent analyses controlled for SES effects by using the regressed residuals of SES and adjustment outcomes variables.

*Measures*
Psychological Outcomes
*The Children's Depression Inventory (CDI).* The CDI [Kovacs, 1988] was designed to assess depressive symptoms in emotional, cognitive, psychomotor, and motivational domains by presenting children with sentences describing various levels of depression in children aged 7–17 years. The instrument is typically used to study child depression in relation to social adjustment [Aluja & Blanch, 2002]. Children are asked to indicate the sentences that best describe the way they have been feeling over the past 2 weeks. Each item can be scored from 0 to 2, ranging from a 'very seldom' to a 'very frequent' presence of a given feeling. The total score varies from 0 to 54 points, with higher scores indicating poorer adjustment, and thus, a greater degree of depressive symptoms. Scores of 12/13 or greater are considered to be indicative of significant levels of depression. The CDI has shown good test-retest reliability and internal consistency across various ethnic groups of children [Frigerio, Pesenti, Molteni, Snider & Battaglia, 2001; Twenge & Nolen-Hoeksema, 2002]. In the present investigation, the question concerning suicidal tendencies was excluded, following previous considerations about its inappropriateness in a classroom setting [Santalahti et al., 2008; Samm et al., 2008]. Internal consistency coefficients calculated through Cronbach's alpha for the present sample as well as for separate ethnic groups are reported in table 1.

Social Outcomes
*The Childhood Social Adjustment Capacity Indicators Questionnaire-Self Report (CSACIQ-SR).* This questionnaire [Caprara, Pastorelli, Barbaranelli & Vallone, 1992] was used to measure social adjustment in school-aged children. It has been standardized in Italy and consists of three subscales representing three indicators of a child's ability to adequately interact in social contexts: (a) the emotional instability scale measures child's tendency to experience vulnerability, poor emotional and behavioral self-control (e.g. insulting, spitting, being impolite); (b) the prosocial behavior scale concerns helpful behavior, and social involvement (e.g. enjoying being in the company of friends and classmates, helping others do their homework), and (c) the aggressive behavior subscale evaluates a child's tendency to harm peers or friends physically or verbally (e.g. fighting with others, saying bad words).

The operational definition of emotional instability as a distinctive social behavior from aggression was adopted from Caprara et al. [1992]. More specifically, this variable has been referred to a particular child's behavior denoting lack of adequate self-control due to a tendency to react impulsively, controversially or rudely in social situations [Caprara et al., 1992]. Higher emotional instability and aggression scores and lower prosocial behavior scores indicate higher difficulties in children's adjustment. Studies have confirmed good psychometric qualities of the scales [Caprara & Pastorelli, 1993; Caprara, Barbaranelli, Pastorelli, Cermak & Rosza, 2001]. Internal consistency coefficients for the present sample as well as for the four ethnic groups are reported in table 1.

*The Childhood Social Adjustment Capacity Indicators Questionnaire-Teacher Report (CSACIQ-TR).* This measure [Caprara et al., 1992] is parallel to the self-report form. Using a 3-point Likert scale, teachers were asked to indicate how frequently a target child showed behaviors such as being rude, threatening others, enjoying being in the company of friends and classmates. The manual reports satisfactory psychometric properties of the scales in terms of construct validity for emotional instability (alpha = 0.94), prosocial behavior (alpha = 0.91), and aggression (alpha = 0.93) [Caprara et al., 1992].

*Procedure*
Based on municipal data from three main cities in Northeastern Italy (Trieste, Udine and Pordenone), schools with high densities of immigrant students were selected for participation in the study. After obtaining signed permission from principals and teachers' councils, participating schools provided access to students and teachers. Bilingual Albanian, Serbian and Slovene research assistants described the project to teachers and requested their involvement. Parents were sent a letter with a description of the project and informed signed consent was collected. Because all children attended Italian schools, the questionnaires were presented in Italian.

All immigrant children were able to speak Italian fluently enough to fill in the questionnaires in that language. Additionally, supervision and support in the interview setting was provided, as all self-report measures were individually administered to each child in a separate room provided by the schools. Children's teachers filled out the CSACIQ-TR [Caprara et al., 1992] individually. Because of a high teacher non-response rate (56%), the CSACIQ-TR could only be administered to a subsample of children (n = 358). There were no significant group differences in social adjustment problems between children with and without teacher reports.

# Results

Prior to conducting analysis to address the main research questions, the impact of socioeconomic background was explored. Because of ethnic group differences in SES (see table 1), SES effects on the dependent variables were examined in analyses of variance. Self-reported lower SES was significantly associated with higher depressive levels [$F(2, 587) = 5.98, p < 0.003, \eta^2 = 0.020$], lower prosocial behavior [$F(2, 587) = 5.88, p < 0.003, \eta^2 = 0.020$] as well as higher emotional instability [$F(2, 587) = 10.27, p < 0.001, \eta^2 = 0.034$] and aggression [$F(2, 587) = 4.39, p < 0.013, \eta^2 = 0.015$]. All subsequent analyses controlled for these effects by using the regressed residuals of SES and adjustment variables.

According to teacher reports, children with lower SES showed lower levels of prosocial behavior [$F(2, 330) = 4.21, p < 0.001, \eta^2 = 0.025$], whereas there were no differences in emotional instability [$F(2, 330) = 1.38, p = 0.252, \eta^2 = 0.008$] or aggression [$F(2, 330) = 1.60, p = 0.202, \eta^2 = 0.010$].

In a further step, we investigated the relationship between self- and teacher scores on children's outcomes by running Pearson linear correlations on the three social adjustment variables. Children's self-reports were significantly and positively correlated with their teachers' evaluations: emotional instability [$r(358) = 0.24, p < 0.001$], prosocial behavior [$r(358) = 0.17, p < 0.001$] and aggression [$r(358) = 0.25, p < 0.001$].

## Ethnic Differences in Children's Adjustment Outcomes

All analyses were conducted using regressed residuals of SES on each of the adjustment factors (psychological and social outcomes) as dependent variables, and ethnic group (Albanian, Serbian, Italian and Slovene) as independent variable. Specifically, one 4 (ethnic group) by 4 (emotional instability, prosocial behavior, aggression and depression) MANOVA was performed on self-reports. A second 4 (ethnic group) by 3 (emotional instability, prosocial behavior and aggression) MANOVA was carried out separately on teachers' reports.

Results of univariate test statistics showed that Albanian and Serbian immigrant children reported lower emotional instability [$F(3, 587) = 3.89, p < 0.009, \eta^2 = 0.020$] and aggression [$F(3, 587) = 3.25, p < 0.021, \eta^2 = 0.016$] than their non-immigrant peers, while no differences were found in prosocial behavior [$F(3, 587) = 1.46, p < 0.224, \eta^2 = 0.007$] and depression [$F(3, 587) = 0.92, p < 0.427, \eta^2 = 0.005$]. Conversely, teacher's reports did not show any statistically significant ethnic group differences with regard to the variables of emotional instability [$F(3, 330) = 1.46, p = 0.224, \eta^2 = 0.013$], prosocial behavior [$F(3, 330) = 2.05, p = 0.106, \eta^2 = 0.019$] and aggression [$F(3, 330) = 2.15, p = 0.093, \eta^2 = 0.019$]. In other words, according to children's self-reports, there is an indication of the immigrant advantage in relation to emotional instability and aggression, but not to prosocial behaviors and depressive symptoms, while according to the teacher's reports there are no differences whatsoever between the ethnic groups (tables 2 and 3). Notably, the lack of differences in the above-reported social outcomes clearly points to the fact that both immigrant and minority children present good adjustment levels compared to their native peers.

## Gender Differences in Children's Adjustment Outcomes

Gender effects on psychological and social adjustment variables were examined in analyses of variance in both self- and teacher reports by using the regressed residuals of SES and adjustment outcomes variables. According to self-reports, boys showed significantly higher levels of emotional instability [$F(1, 587) = 20.01, p < 0.001, \eta^2 = 0.033$] and aggression [$F(1, 587) = 22.01, p < 0.001, \eta^2 = 0.036$] and lower levels of prosocial behavior [$F(1, 587) = 27.65, p < 0.001, \eta^2 = 0.045$] than girls. No significant gender effects emerged

**Table 2.** Self-reports on children's adjustment according to ethnic group and gender (SES controlled by using regressed residuals of SES)[a]

| Adjustment | Total | | Albanian | | Slovene | | Italian | | Ethnicity | | Gender | | Ethnicity × gender | |
|---|---|---|---|---|---|---|---|---|---|---|---|---|---|---|
| | boys | girls | boys | girls | boys | girls | boys | girls | F | $\eta^2$ | F | $\eta^2$ | F | $\eta^2$ |
| Emotional instability | 19.35 (4.13) | 17.63 (4.10) | 18.81 (3.47) | 16.21 (4.10) | 18.58 (3.97) | 18.34 (4.19) | 19.88 (4.49) | 18.73 (3.94) | 3.89**,b | 0.020 | 20.01**,c | 0.033 | 2.22 | 0.011 |
| Prosocial behavior | 20.13 (2.68) | 21.22 (2.52) | 19.90 (2.76) | 21.48 (2.10) | 20.03 (2.72) | 21.41 (2.99) | 20.57 (2.60) | 21.36 (2.40) | 1.46 | 0.007 | 27.65**,c | 0.045 | 0.506 | 0.003 |
| Aggression | 14.69 (4.07) | 13.18 (3.42) | 13.53 (3.42) | 12.13 (3.23) | 14.39 (3.18) | 14.22 (3.78) | 15.12 (4.41) | 13.80 (3.48) | 3.25*,b | 0.016 | 22.01**,c | 0.036 | 1.08 | 0.016 |
| Depression | 10.02 (6.06) | 9.26 (5.65) | 10.79 (5.20) | 9.19 (4.87) | 8.35 (5.68) | 8.69 (7.11) | 9.57 (6.78) | 8.78 (5.93) | 0.92 | 0.005 | 1.05 | 0.002 | 0.365 | 0.002 |

* $p < 0.05$. ** $p < 0.001$. Values are expressed as mean (SD).
[a] Similar results are obtained by considering the interaction of SES and ethnicity.
[b] Refers to significant group comparison between immigrant (Albanian and Serbian) and native (Italian and Slovene) groups.
[c] Refers to significant gender comparison between boys and girls.

**Table 3.** Teacher reports on children's adjustment according to ethnic group and gender (SES controlled by using regressed residuals of SES)[a]

| Adjustment | Total | | Albanian | | Slovene | | Italian | | Ethnicity | | Gender | | Ethnicity × gender | |
|---|---|---|---|---|---|---|---|---|---|---|---|---|---|---|
| | boys | girls | boys | girls | boys | girls | boys | girls | F | $\eta^2$ | F | $\eta^2$ | F | $\eta^2$ |
| Emotional instability | 18.80 (5.50) | 15.89 (4.56) | 18.26 (5.28) | 15.57 (4.48) | 20.37 (4.50) | 16.59 (3.63) | 18.91 (6.25) | 13.92 (4.93) | 1.46 | 0.013 | 26.86*,b | 0.075 | 0.037 | 0.000 |
| Prosocial behavior | 18.65 (2.97) | 19.97 (2.78) | 18.03 (3.15) | 20.13 (2.34) | 17.67 (2.43) | 19.76 (2.53) | 19.18 (3.22) | 20.21 (3.03) | 2.05 | 0.019 | 18.97*,b | 0.055 | 0.795 | 0.007 |
| Aggression | 12.94 (4.36) | 10.43 (3.26) | 12.03 (3.47) | 10.23 (3.27) | 14.85 (4.32) | 10.45 (2.78) | 13.25 (4.86) | 10.56 (3.37) | 2.15 | 0.019 | 33.45*,b | 0.092 | 0.975 | 0.009 |

* $p < 0.001$. Values are expressed as mean (SD).
[a] Similar results are obtained by considering the interaction of SES and ethnicity.
[b] Refers to significant gender comparison between boys and girls.

on depressive symptoms [$F(1, 587) = 1.05$, $p = 0.305$, $\eta^2 = 0.002$]. Overall, these results are in line with the expectation that boys would show more adjustment problems.

In the next step, we reran the analysis by using teachers' scores to see whether they might show a similar picture regarding the impact of gender on children's social adjustment, again using the regressed residuals of SES and social outcomes variables. The same results as in self-reports emerged in teacher's evaluations, who registered higher scores for boys on emotional instability [$F(1, 330) = 26.86$, $p < 0.001$, $\eta^2 = 0.075$], aggression [$F(1, 330) = 33.45$, $p < 0.001$, $\eta^2 = 0.092$] and lower on prosocial behavior [$F(1, 330) = 18.97$, $p < 0.001$, $\eta^2 = 0.055$] than girls. There were no significant interaction effects of gender and ethnic group either in self- or in teacher reports.[1]

## Discussion

Although the body of studies on immigrant populations in Europe is growing, there is still a lack of research addressing immigrant children with different degrees of integration to the host society, especially in the prepubertal ages. The present paper adds to the existing literature, because it is the first that examined Albanian and Serbian immigrant in comparison with Slovene and Italian mainstream children in Italy. Apart from investigating these ethnic groups for the first time, it also included self- and teacher reports by addressing two main research questions: (1) how does immigration affect the psychological and social outcomes of children, and (2) how is this relationship affected by gender and ethnic background?

What we found with respect to social adjustment indicates that positive outcomes in immigrant populations coexist with disadvantaged social circumstances. Consistent with prior evidence on the selective migration hypothesis, our findings support the notion that migration does not always lead to increased levels of adjustment problems. This finding is in line with prior work, which suggests that although they belong to a population considered to be exposed to higher acculturation risk, some immigrants manage to adjust well and are sometimes even better adjusted than the native population – a phenomenon known as the immigrant paradox [García Coll and Marks, 2009, in press; Sam et al., 2008]. In contrast to the selective migration hypothesis [Fichter et al., 2004], some evidence for the paradox is found even accounting for the role of poor SES in relation to better adaptation outcomes in immigrant children when compared to their native peers. Accordingly, a study using data from nationally representative sample of 13,470 Canadian children between 4 and 11 years found that although immigrant children were twice likely to experience family poverty compared to the native children, they showed lower levels of emotional and behavioral problems and higher levels of school performance [Georgiades et al., 2007].

Our results extend previous research on the relation between socioeconomic disadvantage and well-being in immigrant groups, showing that such relation could portray similar findings in Northeast Italy. Accordingly, Albanian and Serbian immigrant children report lower emotional instability and aggression than their Italian and Slovene peers; this is not the case for variables of prosocial behavior and depression, where immigrant children and their native peers showed similar levels of adjustment.

In other words, immigrant children report better social outcomes (emotional instability and aggression) than their nonimmigrant peers, whereas levels of psychological adjustment (depressive symptoms) are comparable in both groups. One possible explanation might be related to different developmental courses in adaptation domains, with psychological outcomes being more positive in recent immigration to the host country, whereas social and cultural problems showing linear decrease over time. Moreover, the positive outcomes in immigrant children are more likely to emerge for the academic and behavioral, rather than for the psychological domain of adaptation [Sam et al., 2008], although some evidence

---

[1] The same analysis using immigrant and native group comparison yielded only one significant interaction effect of gender and immigrant status. According to children's self reports, immigrant girls registered lower levels of emotional instability than native girls, $F(3, 587) = 5.63$, $p < 0.01$, $\eta^2 = 0.010$.

suggests the opposite [Harker, 2001]. This calls for more caution in discussing optimal outcomes in immigrant populations, which might not be universally applied to all aspects of adjustment or all ethnic groups, thus making generalizations more difficult.

The dissimilarity between social and psychological adjustment outcomes might also refer to a domain specificity of acculturation outcomes [Bornstein & Cote, 2010]. Social and psychological behaviors in immigrant populations have been shown to diverge across different circumstances and situations. Immigrant children may tend to adapt better in social domains of adjustment because they develop successful relationships within their school and peer contexts [Georgiadas et al., 2007]. Accordingly, Sam et al. [2008] report mixed results regarding different domains of adaptation of immigrant youth in Europe. Whereas an immigrant advantage was found for the sociocultural domain of school and behavioral adjustment, it did not emerge for psychological outcomes such as anxiety and depression.

Another important issue regards group reference effects [Heine, Lehman, Peng & Greenholtz, 2002]. Social comparisons are primarily made within the same group context and similar others, thus allowing the individual to self-enhance [Collins, 1996]. The perceptions of immigrant children on different adjustment dimensions may be determined by their comparison within the context of Albanian and Serbian national groups, which may be viewed as more disadvantaged and unsuccessful, such that the positive mode of response in immigrant children's self-reports on emotional instability and aggression might depend on their reference group within the host culture. Supportive network of coethnics might serve as a gratifying source of shared experiences, which in turn positively affects individual outcomes [Kosic, Kruglanski, Pierro & Manneti, 2008].

Additionally, our results showing an immigrant advantage for the Albanian and Serbian children's adjustment need to be viewed within the geographical area where the study was conducted. For example, recent study comparing health symptoms and subjective well-being in a large adolescent sample in another Northern region in Italy reports that immigrant adolescents, as compared to natives, are more often affected by psychosomatic symptoms, and are less satisfied and happy about their health and life [Vieno, Santinello, Lenzi, Baldassari & Mirandola, 2009]. Because of its proximity to the Balkan States, the North-eastern region, where our study was conducted, has a longer history of migratory movements from Eastern Europe than the other parts of the country. Starting from the early 1990s, local policies on education and community settings have been adopted to facilitate the integration of these newly arrived families and their children. Moreover, the tendency of stable settlement of Albanian and Serbian groups, as evidenced by high numbers of family reunifications, Italian nationality acquisitions and mixed marriages indicates the presence of an accommodating local community context [Marra, 2002]. All these factors might partly explain positive social adjustment outcomes for children of Albanian and Serbian immigrant families in the area considered.

Although there were weak correlations between teacher and self-reports, findings on group differences regarding children's self-ratings were not supported by teacher reports. According to teacher evaluations, Albanian and Serbian children did not differ from their Italian and Slovene peers in social outcomes. These results are in accordance with evidence from previous studies in which teacher ratings were used to compare immigrant and native youth [Loo & Rapport, 1998]. It is also possible that immigrant children may truly report more positive peer interactions than natives, and it may be that such differences are not perceived in a school setting by their teachers. Moreover, the negative image of immigrant children in Italy may also have another effect, as most of the teachers are aware of Albanian and Serbian stigmatization and low status in the Italian society. Consequently, it is also possible that teachers share the negative societal stereotypes of immigrants in Italian society.

Our results did not reveal ethnic differences in adaptation between the two groups of immigrant children under investigation (i.e. Albanian and Serbian). Interestingly and contrary to our expectation, this result seems to suggest relevant similarities underlying adaptation processes of Albanian and Serbian communities even in the face of substantial differences in culture of origin, history of migration and acculturation experiences in the Northeastern Italy. Irrespective of immigrant status or differences in social position compared to the mainstream population, members of both Albanian and Serbian communities have access to good educational, occupational and health care services. Arguably, the contribution of these factors might underscore similarities in adjustment observed between our Albanian and Serbian participants. Studies in other countries using the same ethnic groups of 7- to 15-year-old immigrant children and youth report mixed findings. Compared to mainstreamers, Albanian immigrant children in Greece were found to experience more behavioral problems [Motti-Stefanidi et al., 2008], whereas Serbian immigrants in Austria have been reported to be less involved in bullying and victimization [Strohmeier et al., 2008]. Such ethnic and immigrant group dissimilarity might be attributable to long-term immigration policies in Austria, compared to relatively recent immigrant flows and consequent reception in Greece, as well as to differences in the adjustment outcome variables used.

Gender comparisons in both self- and teacher reports showed that boys in all groups reported being less emotionally stable, less prosocially oriented and engaging in more aggressive acts compared to girls. Accordingly, these findings are consistent with results from previous studies showing that boys display more aggressive [Derlyn et al., 2008] and socially problematic behavior [Sam et al., 2008] than girls. The current study replicates these gender effects and extends previously reported findings on the relation between gender and social adjustment, by applying them to a sample of immigrant and non-immigrant school-aged children in the Northeastern Italian context.

*Limitations*

Although this is the first comparative study providing some evidence on children's adjustment outcomes in different ethnic groups in Northeastern Italy, some limitations need to be underscored.

First, future data sets must give careful consideration to the measurement of social desirability effects. Children and teacher reports were consistent with other studies and their findings referring to gender, but not to these specific ethnic group comparisons. In addition, the higher levels of social adjustment that immigrant children showed in self-reports were not evident in their teachers' evaluations. By assuming that teachers as external informants are more reliable than children's self-reports, it could be that results on adjustment outcomes might partly depend on immigrant children's social desirability. It is also possible that perceptions of problem levels vary with the informant questioned. For example, Stevens et al. [2003] found that according to self-reports, immigrant compared to non-immigrant children showed lower levels of behavioral problems, whereas teacher reports revealed the opposite pattern. The authors argue that these discrepancies may be determined by immigrant's stigmatization and low status representation, leading to social desirability. In addition, disadvantaged social status and discrimination may be another explanation for our findings, suggesting that the negative image of Albanian and Serbian immigrants in Italy may be responsible for different answering patterns emerged in self- and teacher reports. Further investigations focusing on convergent sources of information, while controlling for social desirability and discrimination factors remain to be pursued.

Second, the study could include teacher evaluations regarding children's social outcomes in the areas of emotional instability, prosocial behavior and aggression, but not their depressive symptoms. Future research should include teacher ratings on depressive phenomena, as teachers have been shown to report higher depressive symptoms for immigrants than for natives [Crijnen et al., 2000], whereas the opposite is found in children's self-reports [Stevens et al., 2003].

Lastly, an important consideration regarding immigrant children concerns mediating factors within family and community settings. We did not consider contextual or mediation processes such as family stability [Harker, 2001], parental emotional well-being [Almqvist & Broberg, 1999], supportive community [Stansfeld et al., 2004] or accommodating school [Beiser, Dion, Gotowiec, Hyman & Vu, 1995], which have been shown to account for optimal adjustment in immigrant populations. Further research should include measures to assess the context-specific variables that possibly are protective for these children.

## Conclusion

From this study, two major conclusions can be drawn. First, self-reports of adaptive outcomes of immigrant children in Italy can be rather different from their native peers. Regardless of ethnicity, immigrant children report better social outcomes than mainstream children – a difference which is not perceived by their teachers. Still, gender comparisons were consistent in both teacher and self-reports showing higher levels of behavioral problems in boys. Therefore, the latter consistency among informants indicates that self- and teacher-reported adjustment outcomes of immigrant children might be influenced by additional factors which were not considered in this study, e.g. social desirability, prejudice, and discrimination experiences. Second, children from two ethnic groups with a different migration history in the host country are surprisingly similar in adaptation. The assumption that Albanian immigrants have to bridge a wider social and cultural gap than Serbian immigrants, leading to more problem behavior, was not reflected in our data. Thus, the process by which some immigrant children succeed in some and not other aspects of social competence as compared to children from the majority group is still not well understood. These discrepant and exploratory results on immigrant status, history or enclave as risk factors for well-being, suggest the need for a more nuanced research approach on adjustment outcomes among immigrant youth. To truly comprehend the psychosocial development of children from different ethnic backgrounds, it is essential to examine the contexts in which they develop in more detail. Further research is needed, for example, to determine whether immigrant children in other parts of Italy are able to adapt successfully and compete on equal terms with their native-born peers. We hope that this study might stimulate further research in that direction.

## Acknowledgements

This chapter is partly based on the doctoral dissertation of the first author who wishes to thank Dr. Maria Tallandini for her support in developing the project and Ingrid Bersenda, Sara Sinozic, Chiara Cardile and Elisabetta Giovannini for their help in data acquisition.

# References

Almqvist, K., & Broberg, A. (1999). Mental health and social adjustment in young refugee children 3 years after their arrival in Sweden. *Journal of the American Academy of Child and Adolescent Psychiatry, 38,* 723–730.

Aluja, A., & Blanch, A. (2002). The children depression inventory as predictor of social and scholastic competence. *European Journal of Psychological Assessment, 18,* 259–274.

Arends-Tóth, J.V., & van de Vijver, F.J.R. (2006). Issues in conceptualization and assessment of acculturation. In M.H. Bornstein & L.R. Cote (Eds.), *Acculturation and parent-child relationships: Measurement and development* (pp. 33–62). Mahwah: Erlbaum.

Beiser, M., Dion, R., Gotowiec, A., Hyman, I., & Vu, N. (1995). Immigrant and refugee children in Canada. *Canadian Journal of Psychiatry, 40,* 67–72.

Beiser, M., Hou, F., Hyman, I., & Tousignant, M. (2002). Poverty, family process and the mental health of immigrant children in Canada. *American Journal of Public Health, 92,* 220–227.

Bornstein, M.H., & Cote, R.L. (2010). Immigration and acculturation. In M.H. Bornstein (Ed.), *Handbook of cultural developmental science* (pp. 531–552). New York: Taylor & Francis.

Brezigar, B. (1999). Post communist linguistic problems in the North Adriatic area. *Nationalities Papers, 27,* 93–101.

Caprara, G.V., Barbaranelli, C., Pastorelli, C., Cermak, I., & Rosza, S. (2001). Facing guilt: Role of negative affectivity, need for reparation and fear of punishment in leading to prosocial behaviour and aggression. *European Journal of Personality, 15,* 219–237.

Caprara, G.V., & Pastorelli, C. (1993). Early emotional instability, prosocial behaviour, and aggression: Some methodological aspects. *European Journal of Personality, 7,* 19–36.

Caprara, G.V., Pastorelli, C., Barbaranelli, C., & Vallone, R. (1992). *Indicatori della capacità di adattamento sociale in età evolutiva.* Firenze: Organizzazioni Speciali.

Caritas e Migrantes. (2009). *Immigrazione: Dossier statistico 2009.* Rome: Anterem.

Collins, R.L. (1996). For better or worse: The impact of upward social comparison on self-evaluations. *Psychological Bulletin, 119,* 51–69.

Crijnen, A.A.M., Bengi-Arslan, L., & Verhulst, F.C. (2000). Teacher-reported problem behavior in Turkish immigrant and Dutch children: A cross-cultural comparison. *Acta Psychiatrica Scandinavica, 102,* 439–444.

Derluyn, I., & Broekaert, E. (2007). Different perspectives on emotional and behavioural problems in unaccompanied refugee children and adolescents. *Ethnicity and Health, 12,* 141–162.

Derluyn, I., Broekaert, E., & Schuyten, G. (2008). Emotional and behavioural problems in migrant adolescents in Belgium. *European Child and Adolescent Psychiatry, 17,* 54–62.

Fichter, M.M., Xepapadakos, F., Quadflieg, N., Georgopoulou, E., & Fthenakis, W.E. (2004). A comparative study of psychopathology in Greek adolescents in Germany and in Greece in 1980 and 1998 – 18 years apart. *European Archives of Psychiatry and Clinical Neuroscience, 254,* 27–35.

Frigerio, A., Pesenti, S., Molteni, M., Snider, J., & Battaglia, M. (2001). Depressive symptoms as measured by the CDI in a population of northern Italian children. *European Psychiatry, 16,* 33–37.

Fuligni, A.J. (1997). The academic achievement of adolescents from immigrant families: The roles of family background, attitudes, and behavior. *Child Development, 68,* 351–363.

García Coll, C., & Marks, A.K. (in press). *Is becoming an American a developmental risk?* Washington: American Psychological Association.

García Coll, C., & Marks, A.K. (2009). *Immigrant stories: Ethnicity and academics in middle childhood.* New York: Oxford University Press.

García Coll, C., & Szalacha, L. (2004). The multiple contexts of middle childhood. *The Future of Children, 14,* 81–97. Retrieved from http://futureofchildren.org.

Georgiades, K., Boyle, M., & Duku, E. (2007). Contextual influences on children's mental health and school performance: The moderating effects of family immigrant status. *Child Development, 78,* 1572–1591.

Harker, K. (2001). Immigrant generation, assimilation, and adolescent psychological well-being. *Social Forces, 79,* 969–1004.

Heine, S.J., Lehman, D.R., Peng, K., & Greenholtz, J. (2002). What's wrong with cross-cultural comparisons of subjective Likert scales? The reference-group effect. *Journal of Personality and Social Psychology, 82,* 903–918.

Holmberg, L.I., & Hellberg, D. (2008). Characteristics of relevance for health in Turkish and Middle Eastern adolescent immigrants compared to Finnish immigrants and ethnic Swedish teenagers. *The Turkish Journal of Paediatrics, 50,* 418–425.

Janssen, M.M.M., Verhulst, F.C., Bengi-Arslan, L., Erol, N., Salter, C.J., & Crijnen, A.A.M. (2004). Comparison of self-reported emotional and behavioral problems in Turkish immigrant, Dutch and Turkish adolescents. *Social Psychiatry and Psychiatric Epidemiology, 39,* 133–140.

King, R., & Mai, N. (2009). Italophilia meets Albanophobia: Paradoxes of asymmetric assimilation and identity processes among Albanian immigrants in Italy. *Ethnic and Racial Studies, 32,* 117–138.

Klimidis, S., Stuart, G., Minas, I.H., & Ata, A.W. (1994). Immigrant status and gender effects on psychopathology and self-concept in adolescents: A test of the migration-morbidity hypothesis. *Comprehensive Psychiatry, 35,* 393–404.

Kosic, A., Kruglanski, A.W., Pierro, A., & Manneti, L. (2008). The social cognition of immigrants' acculturation: Effects of the need for closure and the reference group at entry. *Journal of Personality and Social Psychology, 86,* 796–813.

Kovacs, M. (1988). *Children's Depression Inventory (CDI).* Firenze: Organizzazioni Speciali.

Leavey, G., Hollins, K., King, M., Barnes, J., Papadopoulos, C., & Grayson, K. (2004). Psychological disorder amongst refugee and migrant schoolchildren in London. *Social Psychiatry and Psychiatric Epidemiology, 39,* 191–195.

Loo, S.K., & Rapport, M.D. (1998). Ethnic variations in children's problem behaviors: A cross-sectional, developmental study of Hawaii school children. *Journal of Child Psychology and Psychiatry, 39,* 567–575.

Mai, N., & Schwandner-Sievers, S. (2003). Albanian migration and new transnationalisms. *Journal of Ethnic and Migration Studies, 29,* 939–948.

Marra, C. (2002). Il monitoraggio dei fenomeni migratori nel Friuli-Venezia Giulia. Una rassegna bibliografica. *Studi Emigrazione, 147,* 702–711.

Motti-Stefanidi, F., Pavlopoulos, V., Obradovi J., Dalla, M., Takis, N., Papathanassiou, A., & Masten, A. S. (2008). Immigration as a risk factor for adolescent adaptation in Greek urban schools. *European Journal of Developmental Psychology, 5,* 235 – 261.

National Statistic Institute (2010). *Annuario statistico immigrazione.* Retrieved from www.regione.fvg.it/statistica.

Portes, A., & Rumbaut, R.G. (2001). *Legacies: The story of the immigrant second generation.* Berkeley: University of California Press.

Sam, D.L., Vedder, P., Liebkind, K., Neto, F., & Virta, E. (2008). Immigration, acculturation and the paradox of adaptation in Europe. *European Journal of Developmental Psychology, 5,* 138–158.

Samm, A., Varnik, A., Tooding, L-M., Sisask, M., Kolves, K., & von Knorring, A-L. (2008). Children's Depression Inventory in Estonia. Single items and factor structure by age and gender. *European Child and Adolescent Psychiatry, 17,* 162–170.

Santalahti, P., Sourander, A., Aromaa, M., Helenius, H., Ikaheimo, K., & Piha, J. (2008). Victimization and bullying among 8-year-old Finnish children. A 10-year comparison of rates. *European Child and Adolescent Psychiatry, 17,* 463–472.

Scarnera, C. (2001). *Istituto nazionale di statistica classificazione delle occupazioni.* Rome: Ruggiero Srl.

Slodnjak, V., Kos, A., & Yule, W. (2002). Depression and parasuicide in refugee and Slovenian adolescents. *The Journal of Crisis Intervention and Suicide Prevention, 23,* 127–132.

Stansfeld, S.A., Haines, M.M., Head, J.A., Bhui, K., Viner, R., Taylor, S.J.C., Hillier, S., Klineberg, E., & Booy, R. (2004). Ethnicity, social deprivation and psychological distress in adolescents. *British Journal of Psychiatry, 185,* 233–238.

Stevens, G.W.J. M., Pels, T., Bengi-Arslan, L, Verhulst, F.C., Vollebergh, W.A.M., & Crijnen, A.A.M. (2003). Parent, teacher and self reported problem behavior in the Netherlands: Comparing Moroccan immigrant with Dutch and with Turkish immigrant children and adolescents. *Social Psychiatry and Psychiatric Epidemiology, 38,* 576–585.

Strohmeier, D., Spiel, C., & Gradinger, P. (2008). Social relationships in multicultural schools: Bullying and victimization. *European Journal of Developmental Psychology, 5,* 262–285.

Twenge, J.M., & Nolen-Hoeksema, S. (2002). Age, gender, race, socio-economic status and birth cohort differences on Children's Depression Inventory: A meta-analysis. *Journal of Abnormal Psychology, 111,* 578–588.

van de Vijver, F., Hofer, J., & Chasiotis, A. (2010). Methodological aspects of cross-cultural developmental studies. In M. Bornstein (Ed.), *Handbook of Cross-cultural Developmental Science* (pp. 21–37). Mahwah: Erlbaum.

Vieno, A., Santinello, M., Lenzi, M., Baldassari, D., & Mirandola, M. (2009). Health status in immigrants and native early adolescents in Italy. *Journal of Community Health, 34,* 181–187.

Radosveta Dimitrova
Department of Cross-Cultural Psychology, Tilburg University
PO Box 90153
Tilburg 5000 LE (The Netherlands)
E-Mail R.Dimitrova@uvt.nl

# Ethnic Identity, Acculturation Orientations, and Psychological Well-Being among Adolescents of Immigrant Background in Kenya

Amina Abubakar[a,b] · Fons J.R. van de Vijver[a,c] · Lubna Mazrui[d] · Josephine Arasa[e] · Margaret Murugami[d]

[a]Tilburg University, Tilburg, and [b]Utrecht University, Utrecht, The Netherlands; [c]North-West University, Potchefstroom, South Africa; [d]Kenyatta University, and [e]United States International University-Africa, Nairobi, Kenya

## Abstract

The aim of the present study was to evaluate the relationship of ethnic identity and acculturation strategies with psychological well-being among adolescents with an immigrant background in Kenya. A total of 269 adolescents from five high schools were involved. The sample included adolescents from Asian, Arab, and Somali immigrant backgrounds alongside native-born. A wide set of measures including the Multigroup Ethnic Identity Measure, Measure of Acculturation Orientation, Social Demographic Questionnaire, General Health Questionnaire and the Brief Students Multi-Dimensional Life Satisfaction Scale were administered. Ethnic identity (particularly the subscale on sense of ethnic belonging) was positively correlated with life satisfaction and psychological well-being. Moreover, cultural orientation towards the country of origin was closely related to psychological well-being. In conclusion, ethnic identity was associated with better psychological well-being among Kenyan adolescents. Conceptual models developed in the West can be applied in the African context when both sociocultural and economic factors are taken into consideration.

Copyright © 2012 S. Karger AG, Basel

Two concepts that are salient in multicultural groups play a central role in this study. The first is ethnic identity, which can be defined as the attitudes towards and feelings of belonging to an ethnic group [Phinney, 1992]. The second is acculturation strategies, which can be defined as the set of attitudes and behaviors that are adopted by immigrants to deal with their ethnic culture and the mainstream culture [Arends-Tóth & Van de Vijver, 2006]. Both ethnic identity and acculturation strategies play a salient role in ensuring optimal psychological well-being among immigrant or minority background [Bals, Turi, Skre & Kvernmo, 2010; Costigan, Su & Hua, 2009; Smith & Silva, 2011; Umana-Taylor, 2004; Phinney, 1992]. The literature provides evidence to show that ethnic identity and acculturation are positively related to, among other things, educational achievement, psychosocial adjustment of adolescents, self-esteem and life satisfaction [Bhui et al., 2008; Phinney & Alipuria, 1990; Smith, Walker, Fields, Brookins & Seay, 1999; Yip & Fuligni, 2002].

The saliency and impact of ethnic identity and acculturation on psychological well-being are moderated by the social structure and day-to-day context of the immigrant adolescents [García Coll et al., 1996]. Thus, it is of both theoretical and practical relevance to extend studies to as yet underresearched regions of the world so as to be able to build a more comprehensive picture of the dynamics surrounding the influence of ethnicity and acculturation on psychological well-being. For example, there is much literature on the ethnic identity of adolescents of immigrant or minority background [García Coll et al., 1996]; however, we could not identify any study of ethnic identity among immigrants in Africa. The current study aimed at examining the relationship between ethnic identity, acculturation orientations, and psychological well-being of adolescents with an immigrant (minority) background in Kenya, East Africa.

The centrality of ethnic identity is influenced by several other factors in the adolescent's environment. Key among them is the status of the ethnic group with which the adolescent identifies (i.e. if the group is socially or economically disadvantaged or privileged) [Phinney, Horenczyk, Liebkind & Vedder, 2001]. It has been observed that adolescents of immigrant background score higher on ethnic identity than those of mainstream background [Costigan et al., 2009; Grossman, Wirt & Davids, 1985; Phinney et al., 2001]. For instance, Wissink et al. [2008], studying 345 adolescents (115 Dutch, 115 Turkish-Dutch, and 115 Moroccan-Dutch), found that Turkish-Dutch and Moroccan-Dutch adolescents reported higher levels of ethnic identity than their native Dutch counterparts, which is consistent with findings from other Western settings, which suggest that non-dominant groups in western societies have stronger ethnic identities than dominant groups [Verkuyten, 2005]. We therefore expect that also in Africa, adolescents from ethnic groups of immigrant backgrounds will have higher scores on the ethnic identity measures (i.e. they will have a stronger sense of belonging and identification with their ethnic group) compared to their mainstream counterparts.

Research also shows that the effects of a positive ethnic identity on well-being are more pronounced in minority or socially disadvantaged groups than in mainstream groups [Phinney & Alipuria, 1990]. Thus, Martinez and Dukes [1997] observed that White American students have low scores on ethnic identity alongside high levels of well-being. For adolescents from minority or immigrant background in the U.S. such as Hispanics, lower scores on ethnic identity were associated with poorer mental health. The positive effect of ethnic identity on mental health in immigrant groups seems to arise from the fact that ethnic identity may act as a buffer against stigma and discrimination [Mossakowski, 2003; Umana-Taylor & Updegraff, 2007]. Adolescents from ethnic groups with a privileged position in society may not necessarily need a strong ethnic identity because they are less likely to experience discrimination.

Among youth of immigrant backgrounds, ethnic identity issues interact with the acculturation process. Immigrants have to deal with the realities of two cultural influences: those of their country of origin and also those of the host country. In a currently popular acculturation model, this process is said to amount to addressing two questions for immigrants: Do I want to maintain essential parts of my ethnic culture and do I want to adopt essential parts of the mainstream culture [Arends-Tóth & Van de Vijver, 2007; Berry, 2003]? If these are answered with either yes or no, four possible acculturation orientations can be defined. Integration, involving an affirmative answer to both questions, implies a combination of both cultures. Separation involves a desire to maintain the ethnic culture, without an intention to adopt the new culture. Assimilation is the opposite (adopting the new culture and no maintenance of the old culture). Finally, marginalization means that there is no desire to either maintain the ethnic culture or adopt the mainstream culture. The choices of the immigrants are partly influenced by the attitudes and behaviors of the mainstream groups towards the immigrant group; for example, higher levels of discrimination are associated with less integration [Berry, Phinney, Sam & Vedder, 2006]. Similarly, a stronger ethnic support network is associated with more integration [Ait Ouarasse & Van de Vijver, 2004].

The relationship between acculturation and ethnic identity has long been of interest to researchers. Ethnic identity is viewed as a vital part of the acculturation process. Hutnik [1991] emphasizes the conceptual independence of identity and acculturation strategies, and has defined four types of ethnic identity that have the same names as and are defined in an analogous manner to Berry's four acculturation strategies. The conceptual independence of ethnic identity and acculturation orientations has been widely accepted. Yet, different findings on their relations have been proposed. Schwartz, Zamboanga and Jarvis [2007] used identity and acculturation as distinct, though related variables. In a study consisting of 347 Hispanic adolescents, they observed that the relationships of ethnic identity to academic grades and to externalizing symptoms were mediated by self-esteem and acculturation orientations; so, these authors viewed ethnic identity as a resource. In a study on immigrant adolescents in various western countries, ethnic identity was strongly associated with separation from the host culture, whereas national identity was associated with assimilation [Vedder, Van de Vijver & Liebkind, 2006]. These authors combined identity and acculturation strategy measures. Similarly, Arends-Tóth [2003] made a distinction between acculturation in private and public domains; she found that ethnic identity is an important indicator of acculturation in the private domain. It can be concluded that there is support for a view in which ethnic and national identity are treated as orthogonal processes; studies have found strong associations between acculturation strategies and ethnic identity, but do not agree on how these associations should be conceptualized.

**Kenya as a Receiving Community**

Many African countries like Kenya have a long history of receiving immigrants who come both for economic and security reasons. In the late 19th century, Kenya received a significant number of immigrants from Asia who immigrated for economic reasons, and in the last two decades Kenya has received a large number of war refugees from neighboring countries. To the best of our knowledge, there has been no study investigating the experience of children from these communities. Several factors may influence the experiences of immigrants in African countries such as Kenya. One such salient factor is the SES status of the immigrants in Africa. In contrast to what can be observed in the African context, a significant percentage of immigrants to Western countries regardless of their earlier status in their country of origin tend to occupy the lower social strata in their host country. In Africa, immigrants especially those of Arab and Asian origins due to historical factors have been able to build a strong economic and social position that gives them a comparatively high social status. So, even though they may be a numerical minority, their relative wealth allows them to build up social structures for their own community that support them and potentially buffer them against any negative effects of immigrant/minority status. Our theoretical framework suggests that the context of reception is important for the relationship between ethnic identity and acculturation on psychological well-being. There is therefore a need to investigate the experience of the adolescent in this unique and underresearched group. Studies investigating adolescents in Africa provide information about the degree to which conceptual and theoretical frameworks developed in Western countries apply to a different immigration context.

**Kenyan Context**

The Republic of Kenya is a country in East Africa. The country lies along the Indian Ocean to its southeast and is bordered by Somalia to the northeast, Ethiopia to the north, Sudan to the northwest, Uganda to the west, and Tanzania to the south. The largest cities are Nairobi, Mombasa, and Kisumu. Kenya's population is estimated at nearly 39 million, and it is made up of more than 42 ethnic groups. Kenya has a very long history of early settlements and immigration. This is especially true as it relates to the visitors from the Middle East and Persia who come for trade purposes. In the following sections, we briefly discuss the history of the three ethnic group of interest to this study.

*Arab-Kenyans*
Throughout the centuries, the Kenyan Coast has been host to many merchants and explorers. Among the most enduring and influential visitors to the Kenyan coast have been the sailors from the Middle East and the Persian gulf who travelled to the East Coast for trading purposes. Writings regarding the presence of Arab merchants at the East coast of Africa date back at least 2,500 years. Through trading, marriage, and conquest, the Arabs settled at the Kenyan coast several centuries ago. Most of the merchants visiting the East African coast came from Oman, Yemen, and Persia. One of the major influences resulting from these settlements is the development of the Swahili culture and ethnic group. Many city states including Mombasa, Malindi, and Lamu were developed during this trading period. Immigration from the Arab world continues to be active largely for trading, marriage, and family reunification.

*Asian-Kenyans*
Kenyans of Asian origin largely came from India and Pakistan [Herzig, 2006]. They came to Kenya at different times with different reason. For more than 2,000 years, Asians have travelled to the East Coast of Africa for trading. Unlike the Arabs, the early Asian traders did not settle at the East African coast. However, major settlements took place with the coming of the British colonial power. During the colonial period, the Kenyan Asians changed their merchant and trading patterns. At the beginning of the British colonial period, many Asians were brought to work as contract workers especially in the building of the Kenya-Uganda railway line [Herzig, 2006]. The building of the Kenya-Uganda railways was tough and left many of the workers dead; a significant number of those who survived went back to India [Herzig, 2006]. However, with the formal colonization of Kenya, and the official adaptation of the segregation acts which granted Asians more opportunities for middle level jobs, a large number of Asians voluntarily travelled to Kenya to take up middle level clerical jobs or start a business. An important characteristic of a significant percentage of Asian immigrants to Kenya is that they largely come from impoverished rural backgrounds in India, and travelled to East Africa in search of a better life; many succeeded to improve their social and economic status. Many of the Asians settled around three major towns in Kenya: Nairobi, Mombasa and Kisumu. In these and other towns, they mainly live in concentrated areas forming community centers, schools, recreational centers and sometimes exclusive housing apartment [Patel, 2007]. They were therefore able to organize their cultural activities and have a very vital ethnic life. After independence, the status of Asian Kenyans slightly changed. With the official introduction of the Africanization program, many Asian Kenyans lost government jobs and a significant number decided to immigrate to the UK taking their numbers down from 180,000 in 1964 to a low of 80,000 in 1968. However, the Asians who chose to remain in Kenya continued to play a significant role in the economic life of the country having set up both small and large-scale businesses. Asian immigrants continue to come to Kenya for trading, family reunification and marriage purposes.

Recent census put the number of Asians in Kenya at 35,000 people[1].

*Somali-Kenyans*

Kenya has mainstream Somalis population, an immigrant Somali population and Somali refugees. The demarcation line between these three groups is not sharply defined. During the partitioning of Africa into nations, the Somali ethnic group was separated and placed in various African nations including Somalia, Ethiopia, Djibouti, and Kenya. After independence, the inhabitants of the northern part of Kenya wanted to separate from Kenya so that they could join the Republic of Somalia [Mburu, 1999]. These aspirations resulted in a four-year secessionist war and several years of banditry activism popularly referred to as 'Shifta wars'. The instability and insecurity resulting from the war had a costly effect on the development and integration of the Northern part of Kenya (Somali country) with the region lagging behind in infrastructure, education and other social services [Mburu, 1999]. The war and ensuing underdevelopment effectively rendered most of the Somali population a marginalized and underserved community in comparison to other parts of Kenya. The end of the secessionist movement in the late 1970s and early 1980s led to a rise in the fortune of the Somalis, although they still remained largely out of the public domain. The 1991 war in Somalia led to a new influx of Somalis in Kenya. Since the beginning of the Somalia war in 1991, Kenya hosts the largest number of Somali refugees in the world. While a significant number stay in the United Nation provided camps, many have moved into the towns and cities creating vibrant small and large-scale businesses. This has led to a change in both socioeconomic status and the demography of the Somalis in Kenya. Given the existence of Somali-Kenyans and the strong desire for Somali immigrants not to be identified as non-Kenyans, confirming the immigration status of Somalis in Kenya is a challenging task. While there are indications on the number of 'Somali refugees in Kenya', there is no official figure on Somali immigrations. Somali immigrants who are settled in Kenya rarely self-identify as immigrants. The last population census indicated that there were 2,385,572 million Somalis in Kenya[2].

## Ethnic Identity and Acculturation Orientations in These Groups

There is much research that indicates that immigrants are more oriented towards their ethnic culture and will have a stronger ethnic identity if they experience more discrimination by mainstream members [Berry et al., 2006], experience more cultural differences with the mainstream culture [Galchenko & Van de Vijver, 2007; Nesdale & Mak, 2003], and their ethnic community shows a higher ethnic vitality (i.e. when they have more institutions like shops and places of worship that cater for their community [Suanet & Van de Vijver, 2008]).

There are no studies of ethnic vitality (i.e. the extent to which an ethnic groups has organized systems and structures, including institutions like ethnic shops and places of worship, that support the interactions between members of the groups [Giles, Bourhis & Taylor, 1977]) in Kenya. On the basis of our observations in the field stage of this study, we get the impression that all three communities are vibrant and have a high level of ethnic vitality. Regrettably, there are no studies of the cultural distance immigrants experience vis-à-vis

---

[1] This number is contested. It is believed the census heavily underestimated the number of Kenyan Asians due to coding errors. Various factors point to the possibility of this error. For instance, it is reported that Kenya has 53,393 people who are Hindu. Given that mainstream Kenyans are not Hindu, then one would expect that all the Kenyan Hindu are of Asian origins.

[2] The government cancelled the results from the Somali community. This cancellation was based on the fact that given birth and death projections and expected population growth dynamics, it was deemed statistically impossible for the Somali population to have grown from less than 800,000 10 years ago to nearly 3 million.

**Table 1.** Sample characteristics

|  | Arabs | Mainstream | Somalis | Asians |
|---|---|---|---|---|
| Total (females) | 63 (33) | 74 (39) | 46 (29) | 86 (48) |
| Mean age (SD) | 16.38 (1.45) | 16.77 (2.31) | 16.13 (1.57) | 16.27 (1.39) |
| Mean SES (SD) | 4.72 (1.88) | 6.22 (2.00) | 5.33 (0.70) | 4.27 (1.39) |

the mainstream group. Therefore, the classification presented here is largely based on the first author's observations and knowledge about the historical context of these immigrant groups. Somalis are assumed to be the closest to the mainstream because there is a significant number of Somali Kenyans and the Somalis share the black African identity. The second are the Arabs, whose cultural influence and integration into the Kenyan culture makes them closer to several ethnic groups in Kenya and especially the coastal communities. Lastly, the Asian-Kenyans are assumed to have the largest cultural distance since many prefer to live in culturally homogeneous settings and many of them do not have many informal encounters with the Black population.

## Hypotheses

The current study set out to investigate the relationship between ethnic identity, acculturation strategy and psychological well-being of Arab-Kenyans, Asian-Kenyans, and Somali-Kenyans. In keeping with current research, ethnic identity and acculturation are viewed here as (partly or fully) mediating the relation between background variables (age, gender and ethnicity) and psychological outcomes like mental health and well-being [e.g. Arends-Tóth & Van de Vijver, 2006; Berry et al., 2006]. Based on the reviewed literature, we test the following hypotheses:

Hypothesis 1: Kenyans of Asian, Arab and Somali origins have significantly higher scores on a measure of (their own) ethnic identity compared to mainstream groups.

Hypothesis 2: Kenyans of Asian origin have higher ethnic identity scores compared to Kenyans of Arab and Somali origins.

Hypothesis 3: Ethnic identity mediates the relationship between psychological well-being, acculturation and background variables.

Hypothesis 4: Kenyan Somalis and Arabs would have a relatively stronger preference for orientation towards the Kenyan culture compared to Asians.

## Methods

*Site and Samples*
The study was carried out in three major towns in Kenya (Nairobi, Mombasa, and Kisumu). Students were approached in schools following the granting of permission to conduct this study by the relevant authorities. Five schools were purposively sampled. Schools were selected if they attracted a large immigrant population. Purposive sampling is necessitated by the sample characteristics since most immigrants prefer to attend specific schools. A total of 269 of students completed the whole questionnaire. Table 1 presents the sample characteristics (age, gender, and SES) by ethnic groups both for immigrant and mainstream adolescents.

*Measures*
A set of measures aimed at investigating ethnic label, ethnic identity, acculturation, well-being and social demographic characteristics was administered.

*Ethnic Label.* Students were requested to self identify as to which group they belong to. Additionally, we collected data on place of birth for adolescents, their parents and grandparents. Based on this information, we categorized

**Table 2.** Factor loading for ethnic identity measures

|  | Component | |
|---|---|---|
|  | ethnic pride | ethnic exploration |
| I understand pretty well what my ethnic group membership means to me | 0.74 | |
| I am happy that I am a member of the group that I belong to | 0.71 | |
| I feel a strong attachment towards my own ethnic group | 0.70 | |
| I have strong sense of belonging to my own ethnic group | 0.67 | |
| I have a lot of pride in my ethnic group | 0.65 | |
| I feel good about my cultural or ethnic background | 0.65 | |
| I have a clear sense of my ethnic background and what it means to me | 0.53 | |
| I am active in organizations or social groups that include most members of my own ethnic group | | 0.67 |
| I participate in cultural practice of my own group such as special food, music or customs | | 0.64 |
| In order to learn more about my ethnic background, I have often talked to other people about my ethnic group | | 0.58 |
| I think a lot about how my life will be affected by my ethnic group membership | | 0.57 |
| I have spent time trying to find out more about my ethnic group, such as its history, tradition and customs | | 0.57 |

the students into four major groups: Arab-Kenyan, Asian-Kenyan, Somali-Kenyan and Mainstream Kenyans. A cautionary note is that we did not ask for nationality given the sensitive nature of the information. Using these data, we computed generational status for the adolescents. We had two dichotomous scores here, long-term immigrants were those whose grandparents and parents were born in Kenya, while short-term immigrants were those who themselves, their parents or grandparents were born outside Kenya.

*Ethnic Identity.* The Phinney's Multi-group Ethnic Identity Measure (MEIM) was administered [Phinney, 1992]. This is a 12-item measure that investigates sense of pride in and sense of belonging to one's ethnic group. Given that it is a new measure in this population, we investigated its factor structure and internal consistency. As expected, we were able to extract two clear factors, explaining 46% of the variance. Table 2 presents the factor loadings. These factors were similar to what Phinney has reported and are labeled ethnic exploration and ethnic belonging. The alphas for the subscales were 0.64 and 0.81 for ethnic exploration and ethnic belonging, respectively.

*Acculturation Orientations.* A 14-item measure that evaluates the extent to which adolescents of immigrant background enjoy culture, food, and activities of both country of origin and host country was administered. The measure was adapted from previously applied measures [Suanet & Van de Vijver, 2009]. The measure has items exploring both attitudinal and behavioral aspects of cultural orientation as they relate to culture of country of origin and host country (Kenya in this case). Sample items for this scale include 'I like music from my country' and 'I like Kenyan music'. Items were scored on a 7-point Likert agreement scale. The alpha for the two subscales were above the acceptable level, cultural orientation towards Kenya = 0.77 and cultural orientation country of origin = 0.78.

*Life Satisfaction.* The Brief Multidimensional Student Life Satisfaction Scale was used as a measure of psychological well-being [Huebner, Seligson, Valois & Suldo, 2006]. The items in this scale cover five different domains (family, friends, school, self, living environment) and have an additional measure of global well-being. The alpha for the measure was 0.72, indicating a good internal consistency.

*General Health Questionnaire-12.* This is one of the most commonly used self-report measures of general psychological health [Goldberg, 1972]. This instrument was originally developed as a screening test for detecting minor psychiatric disturbance or strain. The measure assesses changes in affective and somatic symptoms relative to usual levels of health, such as feelings of strain, depression, inability to cope, anxiety-based insomnia, and lack of

**Table 3.** Means and SD for variables that predict outcome

| Scale | Arab | | Mainstream | | Somalis | | Asians | |
|---|---|---|---|---|---|---|---|---|
| | mean | SD | mean | SD | mean | SD | mean | SD |
| Ethnic Identity total score | 2.82 | 0.52 | 2.65 | 0.65 | 2.71 | 0.07 | 2.71 | 0.57 |
| Ethnic belongingness | 3.06 | 0.64 | 2.83 | 0.69 | 2.94 | 0.79 | 2.83 | 0.64 |
| Ethnic search | 2.47 | 0.57 | 2.40 | 0.74 | 2.40 | 0.69 | 2.54 | 0.67 |
| General health questionnaire | 9.79 | 6.55 | 10.76 | 6.05 | 8.24 | 4.88 | 11.64 | 6.38 |
| Life satisfaction | 31.57 | 6.31 | 29.53 | 6.82 | 27.98 | 8.70 | 29.33 | 7.55 |
| Cultural orientation Kenya | 35.39 | 8.50 | – | – | 31.80 | 8.94 | 39.06 | 8.06 |
| Cultural orientation country of origin | 37.56 | 6.15 | – | – | 36.48 | 8.69 | 41.53 | 8.50 |

confidence [Mukkaley, Wall, Warr, Clegg & Stride, 1999]. In the current study, a Likert scale scoring procedure of 0–1–2–3 was used for the GHQ-12. A higher score is taken to be an indication of poor mental health. In the current study, the GHQ has an excellent internal consistency with an alpha of 0.81.

## Results

*Ethnic Identity*
Our results indicated relatively high ethnic identity scores in the sample since the mean was closer to the maximum score at 2.72 (SD = 0.59; Max = 4). Table 3 presents the means and standard deviations of the scores per ethnic group. Our factor analysis of the ethnic identity measure identified the two factors found before: ethnic identity exploration and ethnic identity belonging. A paired-sample t test was conducted to investigate if there were significant differences between the reported ethnic explorations versus ethnic belonging. There was a significant difference in the scores, whereby ethnic belonging was higher (M = 2.91, SD = 0.68) than ethnic exploration (M = 2.46, SD = 0.65); t(268) = –10.89, p < 0.001. The significantly higher scores were observed in all ethnic groups. However, these two subscales were highly correlated, r(269) = 0.52, p < 0.001. Consequently, all further analysis used only the summated score, referred to as ethnic identity. A regression analysis indicated that none of the background variables (age, gender, SES, generational status, and ethnicity) predicted the ethnic identity scores, F(6, 262) = 8.94, p = 0.500. The regression model only explained 2% of the variance. These results were inconsistent with our hypothesis since we had expected adolescents of immigrant background to have higher scores on the ethnic identity measure.

*Well-Being and Ethnic Identity.* Hierarchical linear regression was employed to evaluate the relationship between ethnic identity and poor mental health. Step one involved relevant background factors (i.e. age, gender, ethnicity, religion, generational status, and SES). In step two, ethnic identity scores were entered. The same procedure as the one described above was also carried out for life satisfaction. The background variables explained about 10% of the variance in poor mental health: F(7, 261) = 4.07, p < 0.001, age was a positive predictor of mental health (see table 4 for the standardized coefficients). Entering ethnic identity scores added a small, though significant amount of about 2% of explained variance in the prediction of poor mental health, F(8, 260) = 4.24, p < 0.001. In turn, demographic variables explained about 5% of the variance in life satisfaction F(7, 261) = 1.96, p = 0.06 (see table 5 for

**Table 4.** Hierarchical linear regression analyses predicting ethnic identity by background variables (standardized coefficients)

| Model | Step 1 | Step 2 |
|---|---|---|
| *Mental health (constant)* | | |
| Age | 0.18* | 0.18* |
| Gender | 0.10 | 0.09 |
| Arabs | −0.14* | −0.13 |
| Mainstream | −0.00 | −0.01 |
| Somalis | −0.22* | −0.22* |
| Short-stay immigrant | 0.18* | 0.18* |
| Ethnic identity total score | | −0.13* |
| $R^2$ | 0.10** | 0.12** |
| $\Delta R^2$ | – | 0.02 |
| *Life satisfaction (constant)* | | |
| Age | −0.03 | −0.03 |
| Gender | −0.03 | −0.00 |
| Arabs | 0.13 | 0.11 |
| Mainstream | 0.01 | 0.02 |
| Somalis | −0.07 | −0.07 |
| Short-stay immigrant | −0.02 | −0.03 |
| Ethnic Identity total score | | 0.24* |
| $R^2$ | 0.03 | 0.09** |
| $\Delta R^2$ | – | 0.06** |

Ethnicity was dummy coded. * $p < 0.05$; ** $p < 0.001$.

the standardized coefficients from this analysis). Entering ethnic identity scores added about 5% of explained variance in the prediction of life satisfaction, $F(8, 260) = 3.53$, $p < 0.001$. Thus, as expected, a high sense of ethnic identification was observed to enhance psychological well-being.

*Acculturation Orientation*

Only a subsample (n = 110) of the study population responded to the acculturation measure. The acculturation orientation measure was only for students who were first-, second-, or third-generation immigrants; therefore, those who had longer immigration status and mainstream group members did not answer this part of the questionnaire. A MANCOVA was conducted with ethnic group as independent variable, the acculturation orientations as dependent measures, with age and gender as covariates. There was a multivariate main effect of ethnicities on the preferred cultural orientation, Wilks' lambda = 0.87, $F(4, 208) = 3.85$, $p < 0.005$, $\eta^2 = 0.069$. Univariate analyses indicate that there were significant differences in both measures of cultural orientation: $F(2, 105) = 4.07$, $p < 0.020$, $\eta^2 = 0.072$ and $F(2, 105) = 6.40$, $p < 0.002$, $\eta^2 = 0.109$ for orientation towards Kenya and towards country of origin, respectively. A post-hoc analysis indicated that the Asian-Kenyan groups had significantly higher scores than the Arab-Kenyans and Somali-Kenyans on both measures of cultural

**Table 5.** Hierarchical linear regression analyses predicting acculturation outcomes by background variables, ethnic identity and cultural orientations (standardized coefficients)

|  | Step 1 | Step 2 | Step 3 |
|---|---|---|---|
| *Model 1. Poor mental health (constant)* | | | |
| Sex | 0.11 | 0.08 | −0.01 |
| Age | 0.19 | 0.11 | 0.13 |
| Somalis | −0.05 | −0.07 | −0.11 |
| Asians | 0.16 | 0.14 | 0.21 |
| Short-stay immigrants | 0.01 | −0.01 | −0.08 |
| Ethnic identity | | −0.15* | −0.08 |
| Culture of origin | | | −0.31** |
| $R^2$ | 0.07 | 0.09 | 0.17 |
| $\Delta R^2$ | – | 0.02 | 0.08 |
| *Model 2. Life satisfaction (constant)* | | | |
| Sex | −0.19 | −0.12 | −0.07 |
| Age | −0.08 | −0.07 | −0.08 |
| Somalis | −0.33** | −0.29** | −0.26** |
| Asians | −0.28** | −0.24** | −0.28** |
| Short-stay immigrants | −0.23** | −0.20* | −0.15* |
| Ethnic identity | | 0.26** | 0.22** |
| Culture of origin | | | 0.21** |
| $R^2$ | 0.12* | 0.20** | 0.24** |
| $\Delta R^2$ | – | 0.08* | 0.04** |

Ethnicity was dummy coded. * $p < 0.05$; ** $p < 0.001$.

orientation. The results were contrary to our expectations; based on the theoretical framework of cultural distance, we had expected Asians-Kenyans to have the lowest orientation towards the Kenyan culture.

*Well-Being, Cultural Orientation and Ethnic Identity.* Using hierarchical linear regression analyses, we evaluated the relations between ethnic identity, cultural orientation, and poor mental health. The first step involved relevant background factors (i.e. age, gender, ethnicity, religion, generational status, and SES). In the second step, the relevant ethnic identity scores were entered, and in the last step we added the cultural orientation variables. The same procedure as described above was carried out for life satisfaction. The demographic variables explained about 7% of the variance in poor mental health: $F(6, 103) = 1.14$, $p = 0.29$; in the second step entering ethnic identity the explained variance increased to 9%; this increase was not significant, $F(7, 102) = 1.49$, $p = 0.12$. Finally, the third step, where the cultural orientation towards country origin led to the explanation of 17% of the variance, $F(8, 101) = 2.52$, $p = 0.015$. Table 5 presents the standardized coefficients from the analysis. For life satisfaction, demographic variables explained about 12% of the variance: $F(6, 103) = 2.42$, $p = 0.031$; entering ethnic identity in the second step increased the explained variance to 19%, $F(7, 102) = 3.54$, $p =$

0.002. Finally, the third step, adding the cultural orientation towards country origin, led to the explanation of 23% of the variance, $F(8, 101) = 3.95$, $p < 0.001$. Cultural orientations towards Kenya did not predict any outcome. Therefore, our last hypothesis was partially confirmed.

## Discussion

The current study aimed at examining the relationship between ethnic identity, cultural orientation, and psychological well-being so as to critically evaluate existing theoretical and conceptual frameworks in a different immigration context compared to those more frequently studied in the literature. Our results are largely consistent with earlier reports, though there were also important differences emerging in our samples which could be explained by contextual factors.

Based on theories such as the Social Identity Theory and findings from other regions of the world [Smith & Silva, 2011; Wissink et al., 2008], we had expected significant group differences in ethnic identity scores; however, we did not observe any significant group differences in ethnic identity scores across the cultural groups. The lack of group differences could be explained by various factors. However, we most favor an explanation arising from theories of social identity. In these theories, a differentiation is made between 'numerical minorities' and 'psychological minorities'. In this instance, a group that is a numerical minority but still holds a high social status and has a high ethnic vitality may not feel the stigma and pressure that are felt by groups that hold lower status and a numerical minority status. Therefore, the fact that the immigrant groups studied here are a numerical minority but have a strong economic standing and a high ethnic vitality may as well mean that they do not see a need for a stronger ethnic identity beyond what the mainstream Kenyan groups present with. Moreover, the ethnic groups studied here live in largely homogenous communities and do not feel the pressure to assimilate in mainstream communities. It could be argued from a Social Identity Theory perspective that ethnic identity may not be activated in these conditions of group homogeneity and ethnic vitality. So, members of these groups may need to activate ethnic identity as a coping strategy [Tajfel & Turner, 1986] in other situations than we studied. On the other hand, the lack of difference may result from the fact that recent social unrest in Kenya has made ethnic identity a central issue in the nation, thereby raising the scores for even the mainstream group resulting in such high scores that no differences could be observed between them and the immigrant groups. This explanation is strongly supported by the high ethnic identity scores observed in all ethnic groups. On the other hand, we cannot rule out the possibility that ethnic identities were also strong before the ethnic strife started. Ethnic identities were only contested in the public sphere. All groups have a high ethnic vitality and provide a psychologically stable and secure context for ethnic identity formation in the own group. Identification with the own ethnicity has often shown to be strong in various sub-Saharan countries, as exemplified by the high levels of endogamy in many ethnic groups.

The findings on the saliency of ethnic identity for psychological well-being in adolescent populations were corroborated in our study. Consistent with findings from other parts of the world [e.g. Martinez & Dukes, 1997; Matthew & Galliher, 2007], we observed that adolescents with a stronger ethnic identity also had better psychological well-being. We administered two measures of psychological well-being, one of psychological distress and the other of positive well-being. Ethnic identity was more strongly associated with positive well-being than psychological distress. This is consistent with what has been observed in a recent meta-analysis [Smith & Silva, 2011]. These authors noted that 'studies correlating ethnic identity with self-esteem and positive well-being yielded average effect sizes twice as large as those from studies correlating ethnic identity with personal distress or mental health symptoms' [p. 42]. We presume that these results arise from the fact that adolescents of immigrant backgrounds may not experience much ethnicity-related stress. If they would experience high ethnicity-related stress such as frequent discrimination, then they would use their ethnic identity as a buffer, which would then make the relation of ethnic identity and distress stronger. It is probable that the reasons for individual differences in distress in these groups are not ethnicity related, but probably related to other aspects in life (parents, school, friendships, etc.).

In all the studied groups, significantly higher scores were observed on the ethnic belonging subscales compared to the ethnic exploration subscale, which may imply that most of the adolescents committed to a certain ethnic identity with limited if any exploration. This finding fits in a general pattern that the adolescents in our sample do not live in an environment where their ethnic identity is contested, nor do they experience a strong desire to change their ethnic identity. The higher scores on ethnic belonging subscales seem to be those that were closely related to the positive well-being in this population. These results confirm the hypothesis that the experienced 'sense of community' meets the attachment and belonging needs in most immigrants, which promotes psychological well-being. Again, our findings suggest that the adolescents live in an environment in which ethnicity is not a 'hot topic' or a bone of contention; rather, their ethnic orientation is strongly focused on their own group, which provides a secure basis and their ethnic orientation is widely shared within their respective communities and apparently does not require much further consideration.

Our results indicate that there was a main effect of ethnicity on cultural orientation with Asian-Kenyans having significantly higher scores in both attitudinal and behavior aspects of cultural orientation. While the high scores on orientation towards culture were expected of the Asian community, the high score on the orientation towards Kenyan culture was contrary to our expectations, which were based on the cultural distance framework. The Somali-Kenyans were observed to have the lowest scores both on host and original countries behavior and attitude. Further analyses indicated that these results were influenced by length of stay of the adolescent's families in Kenya, and most of the observed differences could be explained by these variables; the longer they stayed, the lower their scores on both cultural orientation scales. The small number of adolescents involved in this study made it impossible to carry out advanced statistics to delineate these issues further. However, the results point to the need of a further evaluation of the issues raised here in a sample that has been selected in a more systematic manner.

Our results highlight the role of cultural orientation and ethnic identity in mental health. Our data suggest that those who were both actively immersed in their culture of origin and maintained a positive attitude towards the host culture (Kenyan) had better psychological outcomes. These findings are in line with what has been observed elsewhere; since it has been reported that immigrants would prefer an integration strategy, as defined in the Berry model, they are likely to have positive psychological outcomes [Berry et al., 2006; Phinney et al., 2001]. As noted by Berry et al. [2006], adolescents of immigrant background need to be encouraged to maintain their cultural orientation as they adapt to the culture of the host country, at least when there is an extensive network of social support and vital ethnic immigrant community like in the present study.

Our hypothesis about cultural distance was not confirmed. Studies in many western contexts have provided strong evidence to support the cultural distance framework [Suanet & Van de Vijver, 2009]. There are several potential explanations for these results. The immigrant groups in Kenya are able to provide for themselves within closely knit neighborhoods in terms of social, economic, and cultural factors. The effects of cultural distance have been previously observed in communities with a low ethnic vitality [Suanet & Van de Vijver, 2008]. It could well be that a high ethnic vitality may reduce the need to interact with members of the mainstream group, which makes cultural distance less salient.

The measure of ethnic identity used in this study was the Phinney MEIM. Psychometric evaluation indicated that the measure retained the same psychometric properties as those reported elsewhere [Phinney, 1992]. To the best of our knowledge this is the first successful application of this version of the MEIM in the African continent. Using a longer version of the MEIM was applied in Zimbabwe, and it was observed that the authors could not fully replicate the factor structure of the MEIM [Worrell, Conyers, Mpofu & Vandiver, 2006]. Further research is warranted to develop more measures that can be used to study the complex nature of ethnicity in Africa.

The current study was exploratory in nature trying out concepts established in western studies in new cultural contexts. The general findings were encouraging. The measures used showed good psychometric properties indicating construct validity and the relationship between the variables were meaningful and largely in the expected directions. However, the study suffered several limitations which may challenge the generalizability of our findings. First, our sample size was small, which led to the construction of larger ethnic groups as opposed to more fine-tuned grouping; Kenya has 42 ethnic groups; as all mainstream members were categorized as one, this may potentially mask significant difference. Additionally, the immigrant and citizen status could not be adequately quantified since students were uncomfortable to give some of the information. Therefore, children were classified as immigrant based on the place of birth outside Kenya of themselves, their parents, or their grandparents. Moreover, all adolescents identifying themselves as Asians or Arabs were classified as immigrants since these ethnicities are traditionally not considered of local origin. Students who did not give information about their ethnicity had to be excluded from the analysis. Our sampling scheme may have made it unlikely to find support for our hypotheses. We used purposive sampling to recruit through schools into this study. We largely targeted schools that had a large immigrant population. The school composition may have had a salient effect on our results especially as they related to cultural distance. Umana-Taylor [2004] conducted a study of Mexican-origin adolescents who were attending one of three schools, which varied in their ethnic composition (i.e. predominantly Latino, predominantly non-Latino, and balanced Latino/non-Latino). She observed that there were significant relationships between the school composition and ethnic identity and well-being. Future studies need to involve more variation in ethnic composition and not only focus on schools with many immigrants as done in the present study.

The relevance of ethnic composition and various other variables addressed in western studies still has to be examined elsewhere. Africa has a long tradition of receiving immigrants. Conducting more studies of ethnic identity and acculturation in Africa will deepen our understanding of the acculturation process, will help to understand what is common and culture-specific in acculturation processes, and will help to design interventions to alleviate acculturative stress and promote positive outcomes in these populations.

**Acknowledgement**

We would like to thank Musili Ikumi, Abubakar Omar, Asya Ali, Newton Mukolwe and Elma Nzai for the data collection, and Khamis Katana for data entry.

## References

Ait Ouarasse, O., & Van de Vijver, F.J.R. (2004). Structure and function of the perceived acculturation context of young Moroccans in the Netherlands. *International Journal of Psychology, 39,* 190–204.

Arends-Tóth, J.V. (2003). *Psychological acculturation of Turkish migrants in the Netherlands: Issues in theory and assessment.* Amsterdam: Dutch University Press.

Arends-Tóth, J.V., & Van de Vijver, F.J.R. (2006). Assessment of psychological acculturation: Choices in designing an instrument. In D.L. Sam & J.W. Berry (Eds.), *The Cambridge handbook of acculturation psychology* (pp. 142–160). Cambridge: Cambridge University Press.

Arends-Tóth, J.V., & van de Vijver, F.J.R. (2007). Acculturation attitudes: A comparison of measurement methods. *Journal of Applied Social Psychology, 37,* 1462–1488.

Bals, M., Turi, A.L., Skre, I., & Kvernmo, S. (2010). Internalization symptoms, perceived discrimination, and ethnic identity in indigenous Sami and non-Sami youth in Arctic Norway. *Ethnicity & Health, 15,* 165–179.

Berry, J.W. (2003). Acculturation: Conceptual approaches to understanding acculturation. In K.M. Chun, P.B. Organista & G. Marı́n (Eds.), *Advances in theory, measurement, and applied research* (pp. 17–38). Washington: American Psychological Association.

Berry, J.W., Phinney, J.S., Sam, D.L., & Vedder, P. (2006). Immigrant youth: Acculturation, identity, and adaptation. *Applied Psychology – an International Review, 55,* 303–332.

Bhui, K., Khatib, Y., Viner, R., Klineberg, E., Clark, C., Head, J., et al. (2008). Cultural identity, clothing and common mental disorder: a prospective school-based study of white British and Bangladeshi adolescents. *Journal of Epidemiology and Community Health, 62,* 435–441.

Costigan, C., Su, T.F., & Hua, J.M. (2009). Ethnic identity among Chinese Canadian youth: A review of the Canadian literature. *Canadian Psychology-Psychologie Canadienne, 50,* 261–272.

Galchenko, I., & Van de Vijver, F.J.R. (2007). The role of perceived cultural distance in the acculturation of exchange students in Russia. *International Journal of Intercultural Relations, 31,* 181–197.

García Coll, C.T., Lamberty, G., Jenkins, R., McAdoo, H.P., Crnic, K., Wasik, B.H., & Vazquez García, H. (1996). An integrative model for the study of developmental competencies in minority children. *Child Development, 67,* 1891–1914.

Giles, H., Bourhis, R.Y., & Taylor, D.M. (1977). Towards a theory of language in intergroup relations. In H. Giles (Ed.), *Language ethnicity and intergroup relations* (pp. 307–347). London: Academic Press.

Goldberg, D. (1972). *The detection of psychiatric illness by questionnaire.* London: Oxford University Press.

Grossman, B., Wirt, R., & Davids, A. (1985). Self-esteem, ethnic identity, and behavioral adjustment among Anglo and Chicano adolescents in West Texas. *Journal of Adolescence, 8,* 57–68.

Herzig, P. (2006). *South Asians in Kenya: Gender, generations and changing identities in the diaspora.* Munster: Lit Verlag Munster.

Hutnik, M. (1991). *Ethnic minority identity: A social-psychological perspective.* Oxford, Clarendon Press.

Huebner, E.S., Seligson, J.L., Valois, R.F., & Suldo, S.M. (2006). A Review of the Brief Multidimensional Students' Life Satisfaction Scale. *Social Indicators Research, 79,* 477–484.

Martinez, R.O., & Dukes, R.L. (1997). The effects of ethnic identity, ethnicity, and gender on adolescent well-being. *Journal of Youth and Adolescence, 26,* 503–516.

Matthew, J.D., & Galliher, R.V. (2007). Ethnic identity and psychosocial functioning in Navajo adolescents. *Journal of Research on Adolescence 17,* 683–696.

Mburu, N. (1999). Contemporary banditry in the horn of Africa: causes, history and political implications. *Nordic Journal of African Studies 8,* 89–107.

Mossakowski, K.N. (2003). Coping with perceived discrimination: does ethnic identity protect mental health? *Journal of health and social behavior, 44,* 318–331.

Mukkaley, S., Wall, T., Warr, P., Clegg, C., & Stride, C. (1999). *Measures of Job Satisfaction, mental health, and job-related well-being: A bench-marking manual.* Shellfield: Institute of Work Psychology.

Nesdale, D., & Mak, A.S. (2003). Ethnic identification, self-esteem and immigrant psychological health. *International Journal of Intercultural Relations, 27,* 23–40.

Patel, N. (2007). A Quest for Identity: The Asian Minority in Africa. Fribourg: Institute of Federalism Fribourg Switzerland.

Phinney, J. (1992). The Multigroup Ethnic Identity Measure: A new scale for use with adolescents and young adults from diverse groups. *Journal of Adolescent Research, 7,* 156–176.

Phinney, J.S., & Alipuria, L.L. (1990). Ethnic identity in college students from four ethnic groups. *Journal of Adolescence, 13,* 171–183.

Phinney, J.S., Horenczyk, G., Liebkind, K., & Vedder, P. (2001). Ethnic identity, immigration, and well-being: An interactional perspective. *Journal of Social Issues, 57,* 493–510.

Schwartz, S.J., Zamboanga, B.L., & Jarvis, L.H. (2007). Ethnic identity and acculturation in Hispanic early adolescents: mediated relationships to academic grades, prosocial behaviors, and externalizing symptoms. *Cultural Diversity & Ethnic Minority Psychology, 13,* 364–373.

Smith, T.B., & Silva, L. (2011). Ethnic Identity and Personal Well-Being of People of Color: A Meta-Analysis. *Journal of Counseling Psychology, 58,* 42–60.

Smith, E.P., Walker, K., Fields, L., Brookins, C.C., & Seay, R.C. (1999). Ethnic identity and its relationship to self-esteem, perceived efficacy and prosocial attitudes in early adolescence. *Journal of Adolescence, 22,* 867–880.

Suanet, I., & Van de Vijver, F.J.R. (2009). Perceived cultural distance and acculturation among exchange students in Russia. *Journal of Community & Applied Social Psychology, 19,* 182–197.

Suanet, I., & Van de Vijver, F.J.R. (2008). The role of ethnic vitality in acculturation among Russian emigrants to France, Germany, and the Netherlands. *Russian Journal of Communication, 1*, 412–435.

Tajfel, H., & Turner, J.C. (1986). The social identity theory of inter-group behavior. In S. Worchel & L.W. Austin (Eds.), *Psychology of Intergroup Relations*. Chicago: Nelson-Hall

Umana-Taylor, A.J. (2004). Ethnic identity and self-esteem: examining the role of social context. *Journal of Adolescence, 27*, 139–146.

Umana-Taylor, A.J., & Updegraff, K.A. (2007). Latino adolescents' mental health: exploring the interrelations among discrimination, ethnic identity, cultural orientation, self-esteem, and depressive symptoms. *Journal of Adolescence, 30,* 549–567.

Vedder, P., Van de Vijver, F.J.R., & Liebkind, K. (2006). Predicting immigrant youth's adaptation across countries and ethnocultural groups. In J.W. Berry, J.S. Phinney, D.L. Sam, & P. Vedder (Eds.), *Immigrant youth in cultural transition: Acculturation, identity and adaptation across national contexts* (pp. 143–166). Mahwah: Erlbaum.

Verkuyten, M. (2005). *The social psychology of ethnic identity*. Hove: Psychology Press.

Wissink, I.B., Dekovic, M., Yagmur, S., Stams, G.J., & de Haan, M. (2008). Ethnic identity, externalizing problem behaviour and the mediating role of self-esteem among Dutch, Turkish-Dutch and Moroccan-Dutch adolescents. *Journal of Adolescence, 31*, 223–240.

Worrell, F.C., Conyers, L.M., Mpofu, E., & Vandiver, B.J. (2006). Multigroup ethnic identity measure scores in a sample of adolescents from Zimbabwe. *Identity: An International Journal of Theory and Research, 6*, 35–59.

Yip, T., & Fuligni, A.J. (2002). Daily variation in ethnic identity, ethnic behaviors, and psychological well-being among American adolescents of Chinese descent. *Child Development, 73*, 1557–1572.

Amina Abubakar
Department of Psychology, Tilburg University
PO Box 90153
NL–5000 LE Tilburg (The Netherlands)
Tel. +31 0 13 4662528, E-Mail A.AbubakarAli@uvt.nl

# Immigrant Youth Adaptation in Context: The Role of Society of Settlement

David L. Sam[a] · Gabriel Horenczyk[b]

[a]University of Bergen, Bergen, Norway; [b]Hebrew University of Jerusalem, Jerusalem, Israel

## Abstract

Using the dataset from the International Comparative Study of Ethnocultural Youth, the chapter examines variations in immigrant youth's cultural identities in three types of societies of settlement ('settler', 'colonial', 'recent-receiving'). In addition, the chapter explores differences in psychological and sociocultural adaptation in the three types of societies and the moderating role of society of settlement in the relationship between cultural identity and adaptation. Results suggest that the type of society of settlement makes a difference in immigrants' cultural identifications and in their psychological and sociocultural adaptation. Immigrants residing in recent-receiving societies where they constitute a small proportion of the larger population and the society has a short history of receiving immigrants generally exhibit low ethnic and national identities relative to immigrants living in settler societies with longer immigration history and where immigrants constitute a relatively larger proportion of the country's total population. Immigrants living in settler societies exhibited stronger majority national identity; they also report the poorest psychological and sociocultural adaptation when compared with their counterparts in the two other types of society. Not only did immigrants living in colonial societies report relatively stronger ethnic identification, they also tended to show the best adaptation outcomes. Not surprisingly, the society of settlement was found to partially moderate the relationship between cultural identification and immigrant youth adaptation. These findings are discussed in terms of how society of settlement shapes the development of cultural identity against a background of attitudes towards cultural maintenance.

Copyright © 2012 S. Karger AG, Basel

One of the major assumptions of cross-cultural psychology sees human behavior as an adaptation to the eco-cultural context of individuals and groups. Variations in behavior are accordingly the result of differences in eco-cultural contexts, and the adaptation thereof [Berry, Poortinga, Breugelmans, Chasiotis & Sam, 2011]. A crucial test of this assumption is the examination of what happens to people when they move from the cultural context in which they were born and raised to another one that is very different. According to acculturation psychology, during cultural change individuals and groups of people may adopt each other's behaviors, languages, beliefs, values, social institutions, and technologies [Sam & Berry, 2010]. However, precisely how and the extent to which this takes place is not clear-cut [Berry, 1997]. Neither is the adaptation that follows the cultural change a straightforward one. Whereas some individuals adapt very well, psychologically and socioculturally, others adjust poorly when compared with either their peers in the society of settlement or their counterparts from the society of origin [Ali, 2002; Beirens & Fontaine, 2011; Escobar, Nervi & Gara, 2000, Suárez-Orozco & Suárez-Orozco, 2001]. As worldwide migration continues to increase, and people move from one society to another, there is growing interest in understanding the dynamics of the resulting adaptation, and the factors that may explain the variations in adaptation outcomes [Fuligni, 1998].

In spite of the widespread assumption that variation in human behavior is a result of differences in eco-cultural contexts, and the central premise underlying the ecological model of development asserting the importance of different settings on human development [Bronfenbrenner & Morris, 2006], there is a dearth of studies that examine how different cultural contexts afford different adaption and developmental outcomes among immigrants of various ages. All things being equal, do some societies of settlement provide better or poorer adaptation to the acculturating individual than others?

It is against this background that this chapter examines how different cultural contexts, specifically societies of settlement, affect the adaptation of young immigrants. In addressing the role that society of settlement may have on young immigrants' acculturation and adaptation, we will try to answer three questions regarding the role of context in immigrants' acculturation. First, does the type of society of settlement affect immigrant youth's cultural identities – the ethnic (minority) and the national (majority) identities? Second, are there variations in their psychological and sociocultural adaptation, that is, does the level of adaptation vary with respect to the type of society of settlement? And, finally, do characteristics of the society of settlement moderate the relationships between cultural identity and adaptation?

To address the above questions, we will be using the dataset from the International Comparative Study of Ethnocultural Youth (ICSEY) project [Berry, Phinney, Sam & Vedder, 2006a]. The ICSEY project was a study designed to answer three main questions regarding immigrant youth's adaptation: *how do* immigrant youth deal with the process of acculturation; *how well* do they adapt, and are there important relationships between *how* they acculturate and *how well* they adapt? Immigrant youth (aged 13–18 years) who are settled in 13 countries (Australia, Canada, Finland, France, Germany, Israel, the Netherlands, New Zealand, Norway, Portugal, Sweden, UK, and US) took part in the study. In all, over 5,000 immigrant youth and over 2,500 national youth completed comprehensive questionnaires. Cluster analysis revealed four distinct patterns (profiles) of how immigrant youth acculturate: *integration, ethnic, national* and *diffuse*.

Briefly, the *national* profile referred to individuals who had primarily a strong orientation toward the new society in which they were living. These individuals also showed high national identity, but were very low on ethnic identity. Individuals characterized by an *ethnic* profile showed a clear orientation toward their own ethnic group; they exhibited high ethnic identity and low national identity. The *integration* profile included individuals who showed relatively highly involvement in both their ethnic and national cultures. These individuals scored high on both ethnic and national identities. Finally, the *diffuse* profile included individuals who seemed to lack a commitment to a clear cultural orientation in their lives. They had low ethnic identity and somewhat low national identity. For a detailed description of these profiles, please see Berry et al. [2006a, b].

The acculturation profiles were found to be related to how well immigrant youth adapted. Immigrant youth with an integration profile showed the best psychological and sociocultural adaptation outcomes, while those with a diffuse profile exhibited the worst; in between, those with an ethnic profile showed moderately good psychological adaptation but poorer sociocultural adaptation, while those with a national profile had moderately poor psychological adaptation, and slightly negative sociocultural adaptation [Berry, Phinney, Sam & Vedder, 2006b].

Even though there is increasing knowledge on how immigrant youth choose to engage in new cultural environments [Portes, 1999; Portes & Rumbaut, 2006], and how these are related to their overall adaptation, much less is known about the impact of the society of settlement on acculturation and on adaptation outcomes. Cultural contexts tend to be multifaceted, and they are likely to vary on numerous components, ranging from distal factors at the societal level such as formal laws of the society, through intermediate positioned factors involving interactions between the larger society and the local members of the neighborhood of residence, to proximal factors within the family [Portes & Rumbaut, 2006; Motti-Stefanidi, Berry, Chryssochoou, Sam & Phinney, in press]. While we acknowledge that the different factors may have varying importance in the adaptation outcomes, we will limit our attention to the relative proportion of immigrants in the different societies of settlement. This variable has been found to be related to various measures of immigrant's adaptation. Veling et al. [2008], for example, showed a relatively high incidence of psychotic disorders among Dutch immigrants living in neighborhoods where their own ethnic group represented a small proportion of the population [for similar results in a British study, see Boydell et al., 2001]. The research evidence, however, is inconclusive; Ryabov [2009], for example, examined data from the National Longitudinal Study of Adolescent Health and showed that immigrant children's educational achievement and attainment were not affected by density and homogeneity of their peer network. We explore therefore this aspect of the society, taking a very broad perspective by looking at the proportion of immigrants in a society as a whole.

Against the background of immigration, enslavement and colonization, we can discern three broad types of societies of settlement among contemporary plural societies. The first are societies that have arisen from colonization, and have since become settlement countries by encouraging large flows of immigrants, on the grounds that immigration is needed for the economic survival of the society. In this chapter, we refer to these societies as 'settler societies'. In our study, this category of society of settlement includes Australia, Canada, Israel, New Zealand and the US. A second category of societies of settlement that includes a number of European countries consists of those that colonized different parts of the world, and have, starting from the period after the $2^{nd}$ World War, given back the colonized countries their independence to some extent. Simultaneously, many of the former colonizing countries have over the years become 'home' for many migrants from the colonies. In spite of cultural differences, many of the newcomers are quite familiar with the cultural traditions of their former colonizers. We refer to these countries as the 'colonial societies', and in our present study this category includes France, Germany, the Netherlands and the UK. Lastly, the third kind of society of settlement is the one we refer to as 'recent-receiving societies'. Societies in this category have a relatively short history of immigration. Many of these countries were emigration countries where several people migrated to countries such as the US. Following the economic boom of the early 1960s, and the fall of such political structures such as the Soviet Union, these societies have started to welcome some immigrants. These immigrants are mostly guest workers, refugees, returnees and immigrants accepted through family reunification. Countries of this type included here are Sweden, Norway and Finland.

Current statistics show that these three groups of societies of settlement differ systematically on the overall proportion of immigrants and the kinds of policies they follow. Based on current figures (see table 1), we find that with some few exceptions, settler societies generally have the highest proportion of immigrants, followed by

**Table 1.** Proportion of immigrants (%) to the national population in the participating countries

| Type of society of settlement/country | Proportion of immigrants at the time of the study (2000) | Current proportion of immigrants (2010)[a] |
|---|---|---|
| Settler societies | | |
|     Australia | 24.6 | 21.9 |
|     Canada | 18.9 | 21.3 |
|     Israel | 37.4 | 25.0 |
|     New Zealand | 22.5 | |
|     US | 12.4 | 13.5 |
| Colonial societies | | |
|     France | 10.6 | 10.7 |
|     Germany | 9.0 | 13.1 |
|     The Netherlands | 9.9 | 10.5 |
|     UK | 6.8 | 10.4 |
| Recent-receiving societies | | |
|     Finland | 2.6 | 4.2 |
|     Norway | 6.7 | 10.0 |
|     Sweden | 11.2 | 12.1 |

We have to acknowledge that these relative proportions are not perfect. While the proportion of immigrants in Sweden at the time of the data collection was almost twice that of the UK, the proportion of immigrants in the UK was almost at par with Norway. Nevertheless, the colonial influence of the UK in contemporary society is far reaching, and therefore we include UK in the colonial societies category.

[a] Most of the information here were retrieved from the following website of the International Organization for Migration on February 15, 2011: http://iom.ch/jahia/Jahia/lang/en/pid/1.

the colonial societies and the new settler societies with the lowest proportions.

Vedder, van de Vijver and Liebkind [2006] conceptualized societies of settlement in terms of the degree of cultural diversity that included proportion of immigrants in the society, diversity policies, ethno-linguistic fractionalization (based on the probability that two randomly selected individuals from one country will not speak the same language [Inglehart, 1997]), ethnic diversity [Sterling, 1974] and cultural heterogeneity (based on demographic factors, such as variations in ethnic origin [Kurian, 2001]). They found a weak or non-significant relationship between cultural diversity and adaptation. Contrary to their expectations, high cultural diversity was generally related to poorer psychological adaptation. Cultural diversity on the other hand was not related to sociocultural adaptation. Of interest, however, was the fact that cultural diversity was meaningfully related to other acculturation processes. For instance, immigrants in countries high on cultural diversity were more positively oriented towards the national group than in countries low on cultural diversity. As Vedder et al. [2006] point out, the combination of a stronger orientation towards both their ethnic group and the national society may suggest that greater diversity provides a salient context in which youth feel able to orient themselves to both groups rather than to choose one. Numerous other studies [see, for example, Nguyen & Benet-Martinez, 2007; Suárez-Orozco & Suárez-Orozco, 2001] have found biculturalism to be beneficial for immigrants' acculturation.

One primary task of adolescence is the formation of a secure, coherent identity [Erikson, 1968], and it has been suggested that inability to accomplish this developmental task can undermine personal adjustment and well-being. As part of their acculturation, immigrant youth are confronted with the task of negotiating a cultural identity in relation to both their traditional heritage culture (ethnic identity) and the wider society (national identity). Research has shown that a strong ethnic identity is related to psychological and social well-being in immigrant and minority youth [Phinney, 1990; Phinney, Cantu & Kurtz, 1997], but findings on national identity are less conclusive. For instance, national identity has been found to predict self-esteem for majority, but not minority, youth. Horenczyk and Ben-Shalom [2001], on the other hand, have found national identity to be related to positive psychological outcomes and better school adjustment among young immigrants in Israel. It is likely that both ethnic and national identities contribute to psychological and sociocultural outcomes in immigrant youth. In this chapter, we explore whether these relationships are moderated by a central contextual variable – the type of society of settlement as conceptualized above.

In acculturation research, adaptation has been defined in a variety of ways, including one's health status, communication competence, self-awareness, stress, feelings of acceptance, and culturally skilled behaviors. In recent years, it has been common to distinguish between psychological and sociocultural adaptations [Ward, 1996, 2001]. The former refers to psychological and emotional well-being, while the latter reflects social skills and competencies required to negotiate a new cultural environment in an effective manner. Van de Vijver and Phalet [2004] sum up these two forms of adaptations as 'feeling well' and 'doing well', respectively. Although the two forms of adaptation are analytically and empirically distinct, they tend to be interrelated. Skillfully managing everyday tasks and maintaining positive interactions with members of the larger national society (i.e. sociocultural adaptation) are likely to improve one's feelings of well-being and satisfaction (i.e. psychological adaptation). Likewise, it is easier to accomplish personal goals and develop positive social relations if one is feeling satisfied and accepted. Following common practices in acculturation research, we will examine both forms of adaptation. Psychological adaptation will be measured in terms of self-esteem, life satisfaction, and psychological problems or symptoms; for sociocultural adaptation, we will be looking at school adjustment and antisocial behavior.

Regarding adaptation, Aronowitz [1984] concluded from a review of the literature that mental health problems were not exclusive to immigrant youth, and that they do not necessarily exhibit a greater incidence of psychological disorders than their native peers. However, immigrant children are at higher risk to develop emotional and social problems because the experience of migration and culture change can exacerbate normal developmental crises (e.g. identity formation). Furthermore, Aronowitz indicated that when young immigrants manifest emotional problems, these tend to be of two distinct types: anti-social behaviors, behavioral and conduct disorders, and identity conflicts resulting in low self-esteem. Accordingly, we focused on self-esteem and behavior problems as two of our outcome variables. In line with positive psychology reasoning [Seligman & Csikszentmihalyi, 2000], we also focused on satisfaction with life, where we wanted to direct attention to more positive aspects of human life.

School adjustment and antisocial behavior were chosen as measures of sociocultural adaptation. The school environment is identified as a socioecological context that is highly influential for youth social development in general; for immigrant youth, schools serve as a major arena

**Table 2.** Demographic description of the sample according to type of settlement society

|  | Society of settlement | | | |
|---|---|---|---|---|
|  | settler | colonial | recent-receiving | total |
| Total participants | 3,078 | 2,035 | 2,522 | 7,635 |
| Females, % | 52.8 | 54.1 | 49.5 | 52.5 |
| 1st generation, % | 32.1 | 10.0 | 32.7 | 27.4 |
| Mean age, years | 15.39 | 15.57 | 15.21 | 15.38 |
| Mean occupational status of parents | 2.71 | 2.50 | 2.18 | 2.48 |

where newcomers learn about the norms, values and traditions of the new society of settlement [Vedder & Horenczyk, 2006]. To acquire the values of the society imparted by the school, it is essential that immigrant children find school attendance satisfying.

In sum, the present chapter focuses on the effect of a central contextual variable – type of society of settlement – on identity and adaptation of immigrant youth. First, we examine variations in immigrant youth's cultural identities residing in three types of societies of settlement ('settler', 'colonial', 'recent-receiving'). We then explore differences among these three types of societies in the psychological adaptation (i.e. self-esteem, life satisfaction and psychological problems) and sociocultural adaptation (i.e. school adjustment and behavioral problems) of immigrant youth. Finally, we explore whether the relationship between cultural identity and adaptation is moderated by the contextual variable under study – namely, type of society of settlement.

## Method

The dataset for this paper comes from the ICSEY project, and a detailed description of the project, data collection, and the samples has been provided elsewhere [Berry et al., 2006a, b]. Only a brief description of the major methodological aspects of the project relevant for this chapter follows.

*Participants*

The immigrant respondents in our study were members of 26 ethnic groups in 12 countries (Australia, Canada, Finland, France, Germany, Israel, the Netherlands, New Zealand, Norway, Sweden, the UK, and the US). The total sample of immigrants consisted of 5,359 adolescents (53% female); 1,538 (32.6%) first-generation youth (not born in the country of residence; 49% female), 3,179 second-generation immigrants (born in country of residence, or born outside, but migrated to the host country before the age of 6, and parents born abroad; 53.7% female). Ages ranged from 13 to 18 years (mean = 15.35, SD = 1.53). On a 4-point scale ranging from 1 (unskilled) to 4 (professional) derived from the combined highest occupation of the father and mother, the mean occupational status of the families was 2.24 (i.e. somewhere between skilled and white collar job). See table 2 for a breakdown of these demographic variables by society of settlement.

Nearly a third of the participants (31.2%) belonged to two ethnic groups – Vietnamese (17.5%) and Turks (13.7%). In addition, the single largest ethnic minority group in the participating countries were Filipino (in Australia); Indo-Canadians (in Canada); Russians (in Finland); Moroccans (in France); Aussiedlers (in Germany); Russians (in Israel); Surinamese (in the Netherlands); Pacific Islanders (in New Zealand); Pakistanis (in Norway); Central, Latin and South Americans (in Sweden) and Indians (in the UK), and Armenians (in the US). The distribution of generation status differed widely in the different countries: Whereas in Germany all the participants were 1st generation, France, the UK and Israel, represented three countries with extreme ratios of 2nd generation immigrants (94.5, 98.8 and 13.2% for France, UK, and Israel, respectively).

Random sampling was not feasible in any of the participating countries. Purposive sampling was used, and this took place at schools, where both the national and immigrant youth attended the same schools.

*The Instrument*

A questionnaire covering a wide range of issues related to acculturation and adaptation was designed for the study by the ICSEY research team (see appendix). For most of the scales, response options ranged from 'strongly disagree' (1) to 'strongly agree' (5). Following is a brief description of the scales in the questionnaire reported in this chapter.

Cultural identities (ethnic and national) were measured using an adapted version of the Multi-Group Ethnic Identity Measure by Phinney [1992] and the scale on national identity developed by Phinney and Devich-Navarro [1997]. An item on the 8-item Ethnic identity subscale was 'I feel I am part of [ethnic] culture', and an example on the 4-item national (majority) identity was 'I am happy to be [national]'.

Psychological Adaptation

Self-esteem was assessed using the scale developed by Rosenberg [1965] with the following as a sample time 'On the whole I am satisfied with myself'.

Life satisfaction was measured using the 5-item Satisfaction with Life scale by Diener, Emmons, Larsen and Griffin [1985]. An example of an item from the scale is 'If I could live my life over, I would change almost nothing'.

A 15-item scale – Psychological problems – was developed by the ICSEY research team to measure depression, anxiety, and psychosomatic symptoms. Two sample items are: 'I feel tired' and 'My thoughts are confused'.

Sociocultural Adaptation

School adjustment was concerned with identifying how adolescents feel about school, and was assessed using a 7-item scale with questions such as 'I feel uneasy about going to school in the morning'. This scale was specially developed by the ICSEY research group.

Behavior problems focused on antisocial behavior, and this was assessed using a 10-item Antisocial Behavior scale developed by Olweus and his colleagues [Bendixen & Olweus, 1999; Olweus, 1989]. A sample item is: 'Purposely destroyed seats in a bus or a movie theatre'. A 5-point response category ranging from 'never' to 'several times in the course of a 12-month period' was used.

All scales had satisfactory to good reliability (Cronbach alphas ranged between 0.70 and 0.85). We examined whether the scales measured the same psychological constructs (i.e. structural equivalence) in all the cultural groups in all the countries using a procedure described by Van de Vijver and Leung [1997]. All scales were found to be unidimensional, and we obtained very strong support for the structural equivalence of the measures across countries [for a detailed description see Vedder & van de Vijver, 2006].

*Procedure*

Data were collected in all countries by members of the research teams (usually postgraduate students or teachers who were often members of the ethnocultural group) who were selected and trained by the researchers in each country.

## Results

The results will be presented according to the three possible roles of context in the acculturation of immigrant youth suggested in this chapter. We will start by examining variations in cultural identities – ethnic and national – among the three types of societies of settlement. Then, we will analyze differences among the societies of settlement in the two aspects of adaptation – psychological and sociocultural. Lastly, we will explore the moderating role of society of settlement in the relationship between cultural identity and adaptation.

A multivariate analysis of covariance was performed first to examine the effect of society of settlement on the z-scores of ethnic and national identities, with generation in the new country (1st or 2nd generation), age, and gender included as covariates. Results revealed a significant multivariate effect of society of settlement [Wilks' lambda = 0.76, $F(4, 9,140) = 337.06$, $p < 0.001$, $\eta^2 = 0.13$]; the univariate effects on each of the two identities were also found to be significant [ethnic identity: $F(2, 4,571) = 18.04$, $p < 0.001$, $\eta^2 = 0.01$; national identity: $F(2, 4,571) = 705.18$, $p < 0.001$, $\eta^2 = 0.24$]. Post-hoc Scheffé tests showed ethnic identity to be stronger in colonial societies as compared to both recent-receiving, and settler societies; national identity, however, was stronger in settler societies, followed by colonial societies, and weakest in recent-receiving societies (see fig. 1).

A second set of analyses focused on the effects of societal context on the psychological and sociocultural adaptation of immigrant youth. Two MANCOVAs were conducted, each including generation status, gender, and age as covariates.

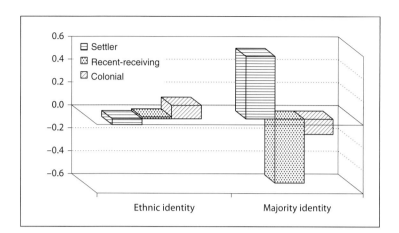

**Fig. 1.** Means of ethnic and majority identities (z-scores) by society of settlement.

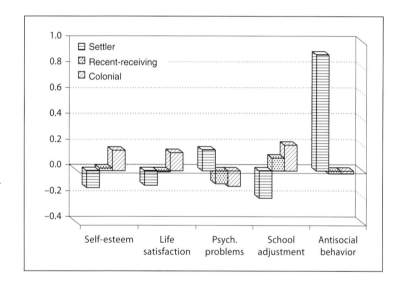

**Fig. 2.** Means (z-scores) of psychological adaptation (self-esteem, life satisfaction, and psychological problems) and sociocultural adaptation (school adjustment and antisocial behaviors) by society of settlement.

For psychological adaptation, we examined the effect of society of settlement on self-esteem, life satisfaction, and psychological problems; school adjustment and antisocial behavior were used to assess sociocultural adaptation (see fig. 2). Society of settlement was found to be related to psychological adaptation [Wilks' lambda = 0.97, $F(6, 8,998) = 23.19$, $p < 0.001$, $\eta^2 = 0.16$] as well as to sociocultural adaptation [Wilks' lambda = 0.94, $F(4, 9,006) = 64.93$, $p < 0.001$, $\eta^2 = 0.03$]. As to psychological adaptation, univariate analyses followed by post-hoc Scheffé tests showed that self-esteem was higher in the colonial societies, followed by new settler societies, and lowest in settler societies [$F(2, 4,501) = 14.04$, $p < 0.001$, $\eta^2 = 0.01$]. Life satisfaction was also lowest in settler societies, higher in colonial societies, and highest in recent-receiving societies [$F(2, 4,501) = 24.56$, $p < 0.001$, $\eta^2 = 0.02$]. Consistent with this pattern, immigrants in settler societies reported more

**Table 3.** Means (z-scores) of psychological adaptation (self-esteem, life satisfaction, and psychological problems) and sociocultural adaptation (school adjustment and antisocial behaviors) by society of settlement and ethnic identity (dichotomized)

| Society of settlement | Ethnic identity | Self-esteem | Life satisfaction | Psychological problems | School adjustment | Antisocial behavior |
|---|---|---|---|---|---|---|
| Settler | Low | −0.43 | −0.23 | 0.15 | −0.76 | 0.05 |
|  | High | 0.08 | −0.03 | 0.16 | 0.16 | 0.11 |
|  | Total | −0.13 | −0.11 | 0.16 | −0.21 | 0.09 |
| Colonial | Low | 0.00 | −0.21 | −0.06 | 0.10 | −0.03 |
|  | High | 0.22 | 0.06 | −0.15 | 0.24 | −0.03 |
|  | Total | 0.16 | −0.01 | −0.12 | 0.20 | −0.03 |
| Recent-receiving | Low | −0.36 | −0.22 | 0.05 | −0.08 | −0.03 |
|  | High | 0.18 | 0.30 | −0.17 | 0.18 | −0.01 |
|  | Total | 0.01 | 0.14 | −0.10 | 0.10 | −0.02 |
| Total | Low | −0.31 | −0.22 | 0.07 | −0.36 | 0.01 |
|  | High | 0.16 | 0.11 | −0.04 | 0.19 | 0.03 |

psychological problems as compared to their counterparts in recent-receiving and colonial societies [$F(2, 4,501) = 45.37$, $p < 0.001$, $\eta^2 = 0.03$].

Immigrants in recent-receiving societies also exhibited worse sociocultural adaptation. Scheffé tests following significant univariate effects [school adjustment: $F(2, 4,504) = 123.05$, $p < 0.001$, $\eta^2 = 0.05$; antisocial behavior: $F(2, 4,504) = 28.17$, $p < 0.001$, $\eta^2 = 0.02$] revealed higher school adjustment and less antisocial behavior in both colonial and recent receiving societies as compared to immigrants in settler societies (see fig. 2).

Finally, we examined the possible moderating role of society of settlement in the relationship between cultural identity and adaptation. Preliminary analyses showed ethnic identity – but not national identity – to be moderately correlated with all measures of psychological and sociocultural adaptation. As expected, higher values of ethnic identity were associated with higher levels of self-esteem, life satisfaction, and school adjustment, and with lower scores on psychological problems and behavior problems. In order to test for moderation, we then dichotomized ethnic identity according to the median, and proceeded to examine multivariate and univariate interactions between society of settlement and ethnic identity on psychological and sociocultural adaptation.

Results provided mild evidence for a moderation effect of society of settlement on the relationship between ethnic identity and adaptation. In both MANCOVA analyses – with generation status, age, and gender as covariates – the interaction between society of settlement and ethnic identity was found significant (psychological adaptation: Wilks' lambda = 0.99, $F(6, 8,968) = 8.64$, $p < 0.001$; sociocultural adaptation: Wilks' lambda = 0.97, $F(4, 8,976) = 39.61$, $p < 0.001$). Table 3 reveals once more the contextual effects of society of settlement, especially with regard to the adaptation of immigrant youth in settler societies. Levels of self-esteem and school adjustment are particularly low, and psychological problems and antisocial behavior relatively high, among immigrants in settler societies who exhibit low ethnic identity.

## Discussion

The results of this study provide additional support for the ecological approach in acculturation research that calls for the examination of contextual effects on various aspects related to the adaptation of immigrants [Horenczyk, 2009]. In this chapter, we have focused on an aspect of the macrosystem [Bronfenbrenner & Morris, 2006], looking at the impact of the sociopolitical system with regard to receiving immigrants on the outcomes of cultural identity and adaptation. Our findings suggest that the type of society within which young immigrants acculturate makes a difference in their cultural identifications, and in their psychological and sociocultural adaptation. In broad terms, immigrants residing in societies where they constitute a small proportion of the larger population as well as when the society has a short history with receiving immigrants, generally exhibit low ethnic and national identities. This is in comparison with their counterparts living in societies with longer history with settling immigrants, and where at the same time they constitute a relatively larger proportion of the total population of the country. Immigrants living in settler societies such as Australia and the US exhibit a relatively higher majority national identity. These immigrants also report the poorest psychological and sociocultural adaptation when compared with their counterparts in the two other societies. In contrast, not only do immigrants living in colonial societies report relatively higher ethnic identification, they also tend to exhibit the best adaptation outcomes. Not surprisingly, the society of settlement appears to partially moderate the relationship between cultural identification and immigrant youth adaptation.

Although we have defined society of settlement on the basis of previous history of immigration/emigration, and the proportion of immigrants in relation to the larger national population, these categories seem to define a dynamic context that helps to shape immigrant youth cultural identity and their adaptation. A key question about our findings is, what is it about the different types of society that shapes the acculturation process to result in high cultural identification in some, and low in others, and how does the level of identity, particularly ethnic identity interact with the society of settlement to result in poor or better adaptation?

The relatively high majority national identity, coupled with relatively low ethnic identity exhibited by immigrants in settler societies can be understood in terms of the perceptions held by the immigrants regarding the host society's expectations related to their cultural identities [Horenczyk, 1996]. Although we have not examined specific settlement policies of any particular country, we suggest that societies pursuing assimilation policies for instance may expect newcomers to weaken their ties to their original heritage culture, and to embrace the culture of the larger society. This might explain this pattern in one of the settler societies included in the study, namely, Israel [Horenczyk & Ben-Shalom, 2006].

On the other hand, we expected that with the relatively large proportion of immigrants in the total population of settler societies, it would be easier for immigrants to retain their original heritage culture [Bourhis et al., 1997]. However, it appears that this is not the case. What we have not examined in the present study is whether the settler societies in our study are in reality perceived by immigrants as following assimilation policies, even if the official settlement policy of countries like Australia and Canada is one of multiculturalism. Policies of multiculturalism are aimed at encouraging immigrants and ethnic minorities to maintain their heritage culture and distinctiveness as they participate in the new society as full fledge members [Berry & Sam, in press]. However, it might be the case that multiculturalist policies and attitudes in some societies are perceived as conveying an open – and relatively warm – welcoming message to immigrants, inviting them to join the larger society with its tolerance to features of minority culture. We suggest that immigrants arriving and settling in these societies may feel encouraged to adopt, as immigrants, an inclusive national identity.

Immigrants living in colonial societies, despite exhibiting relatively low ethnic and national identities, seem to report the best outcomes on the various adaptation indicators we examined. This appears to contradict the widespread claim that high ethnic identity in combination with high majority identity resulting in a bicultural identity is most conducive to successful immigrant adaptation [Benet-Martinez & Haritatos, 2005; Chen, Benet-Martinez & Bond, 2008; LaFromboise, Coleman & Gerton, 1993; Suárez-Orozco and Suárez-Orozco, 2001]. However, the moderating effect of society of settlement on the relationship between ethnic identity and adaptation seems to suggest that the effect of identity on adaption is contingent on aspects of the acculturating context, such as the type of settlement society. As suggested by Phinney, Horenczyk, Liebkind, and Vedder [2001], the role of ethnic and national identities in adaptation should be understood as an interaction between the contextual factors and characteristics of immigrants. Our results showed that the worst adaptation was found among immigrants in settler societies with low levels of ethnic identity.

As indicated in an earlier section, contexts are multifaceted and may include numerous components, ranging from distal factors such as the laws of the society to specific proximal microsystem factors such as the size of the living arrangements [Super & Harkness, 1997]. The path through which the distal macrosystem factor explored in this study – type of society of settlement – translates down to the acculturating individual's adaptation is likely to be complex and to follow a variety of routes. As it is, the observed differences in adaptation outcome could have arisen from one or more proximal factors. Future studies should examine these paths of influence in order to broaden as well deepen our understanding of the role of context in acculturation.

Within the larger framework of contextualized acculturation research, future work needs also to integrate – not only conceptually but also empirically – the variety of contextual factors in order to better predict identity and adaptational outcomes. Factors from different realms of context can be taken into account. Verkuyten [2005] proposed to look into the ideological context, the comparative group context, the cultural context, and the discursive/rhetorical context. The notion of context has been applied both to immediate social situations (such as those in schools and neighborhoods), as well as to larger historical, political, social, and economic conditions [Verkuyten & Zaremba, 2005]. Historical processes have also been emphasized by Deaux [2006] and Garcia Coll and Marks [2009], who argued that immigrants create their life within the historical context, including the migration flow they are part of. The complexity and richness of acculturative contexts call for a long-range research effort aimed at reaching a comprehensive dynamic analysis of immigrants' identities and adaptation.

In terms of youth development in general, this study reinforces the importance of the contextual factors. With respect to immigrant youth, it would appear that the relative size of the immigrant population in the larger society on the one hand helps define the nature of the perceptions of, and the interaction between, immigrants and members of the larger society, and on the other helps shape attitudes within the larger society. The result of this is how immigrant youth define their cultural identity and how it affects their overall psychological and sociocultural functioning.

In this chapter, we looked indirectly at the proportion of immigrants in a group of countries. This manner of categorizing our independent variable places it at a very distal position in terms of effects of contextual factors on adaptation. Consequently, much of our findings should be regarded as tentative requiring further research. Future research should also strive to go several steps further by looking at how cultural identities are shaped by the distribution of immigrant densities in different neighborhood of a country, and how these combine to affect adaptation outcomes. In addition to exploring ethnic densities of neighborhood of a particular country, it may also be important to measure the proportion of immigrants at the classroom level, and explore the effect of context using a multilevel research strategy.

## Appendix

Members of the ICSEY project group are (in alphabetical order of countries) C. Leung, R. Rooney and D. Sang (Australia); J. W. Berry and K. Kwak (Canada); K. Liebkind (Finland); C. Sabatier (France); P. Schmitz (Germany); G. Horenczyk (Israel); P. Vedder and F. van de Vijver (the Netherlands); C. Ward (New Zealand); D. L. Sam (Norway); F. Neto (Portugal); E. Virta and C. Westin (Sweden); L. Robinson (UK) and J. S. Phinney (US).

## References

Ali, J. (2002). Mental health of Canada's immigrants. Supplement to *Health Reports, Vol. 13*, Statistics Canada. Retrieved December 10, 2010, from www.statcan.gc.ca/cgi-bin/af-fdr.cgi?l=eng&loc=http://www.statcan.gc.ca/pub/82-003-s/2002001/pdf/82-003-s2002006-eng.pdf&t=Mental health of Canada's immigrants.

Aronowitz, M. (1984). The social and emotional adjustment of immigrant children. A review of literature. *International Migration Review, 18,* 237–257.

Beirens, K., & Fontaine, J.R.J. (2011). Somatic and emotional wellbeing among Turkish immigrants in Belgium: Acculturation or culture? *Journal of Cross-Cultural Psychology, 42,* 56–74.

Bendixen, M., & Olweus, D. (1999). Measurement of antisocial behavior in early adolescence and adolescence: Psychometric properties and substantive findings. *Criminal Behavior and Mental Health, 9,* 323–354.

Benet-Martínez, V., & Haritatos, J. (2005). Bicultural identity integration (BII): Components and psychological antecedents. *Journal of Personality, 73,* 1015–1050.

Berry, J.W. (1997). Immigration, acculturation and adaptation. *Applied Psychology, 46,* 5–68

Berry, J.W., Phinney, J.S., Sam, D.L., & Vedder, P. (Eds.). (2006a). *Immigrant youth in cultural transition: Acculturation, identity and adaptation across national contexts.* Mahwah: Lawrence Erlbaum Associates, Publishers.

Berry, J.W., Phinney, J.S., Sam, D.L., & Vedder, P. (2006b). Immigrant youth: Acculturation, identity and adaptation. *Applied Psychology: An International Review, 55,* 303–332

Berry, J.W., Poortinga, Y.H., Breugelmans, S.M., Chasiotis, A., & Sam, D.L. (2011). *Cross-cultural psychology: Research and application* (3rd ed.). Cambridge: Cambridge University Press.

Berry, J.W., & Sam, D.L. (in press). Multicultural societies. In V. Benet-Martínez & Y.-Y. Hong (Eds.), *Handbook of Multicultural Identity: Basic and Applied Perspectives.* New York: Oxford University Press.

Bourhis, R.Y., Moise, L.C., Perreault, S., & Senecal, S. (1997). Towards an Interactive Acculturation Model: A social psychological approach. *International Journal of Psychology, 32,* 369–386.

Boydell, J., van Os, J., McKenzie, K., Allardyce, J., Goel, R., McCreadie, R.G., & Murray, R.M. (2001). Incidence of schizophrenia in ethnic minorities in London: ecological study into interactions with environment. *BMJ, 323,* 1336.

Bronfenbrenner, U., & Morris, P.A. (2006). The bioecological model of human development. In R.M. Lerner (Ed.), *Handbook of Child Psychology. Vol. 1: Theoretical models of human development* (6th ed., pp. 793–828). Hoboken: Wiley

Chen, S.X., Benet-Martinez, V., & Bond, M.H (2008). Bicultural identity, bilingualism, and psychological adjustment in multicultural societies: Immigration-based and globalization-based acculturation. *Journal of Personality, 76,* 803–838

Diener, E., Emmons, R.A., Larsen, R.J., & Griffin, A. (1985). The satisfaction with life scale. *Journal of Personality Assessment, 49,* 71–75.

Erikson, E. (1968). *Identity: Youth and crisis.* New York: Norton.

Escobar, J.I., Nervi, C.H., & Gara, M.A. (2000). Immigration and mental health: Mexican Americans in the United States. *Harvard Review of Psychiatry, 8,* 64–72.

Fuligni, A. (1998). The adjustment of children from immigrant families. *Current Directions in Psychological Science, 7,* 99–103.

Garcia Coll, C., & Marks, A. (2009). *Immigrant stories: Ethnicity and academics in middle childhood.* New York: Oxford University Press.

Horenczyk, G. (1996). Migrant identities in conflict: Acculturation attitudes and perceived acculturation ideologies. In G. Breakwell & E. Lyons (Eds.), *Changing European Identities* (pp. 241–250). Oxford: Butterworth-Heinemann.

Horenczyk, G. (2009). Multiple reference groups: Towards the mapping of immigrants' complex social worlds. In I. Jasinkaja-Lahti & T.A. Mähönen (Eds.), *Identities, intergroup relations and acculturation: The cornerstones of intercultural encounters* (pp. 67–80). Helsinki: Gaudeamus Helsinki University Press.

Horenczyk, G., & Ben-Shalom, U. (2001). Multicultural identities and adaptation among young immigrants in Israel. In N.K. Shimahara, I. Holowinsyk & S. Tomlinson-Clarke (Eds.), *Ethnicity, race and nationality in education: A global perspective* (pp. 55–78). Mahwah, NJ: Erlbaum

Horenczyk, G., & Ben-Shalom, U. (2006). Acculturation in Israel. In D.L. Sam & J.W. Berry (Eds.), *The Cambridge handbook of acculturation psychology* (pp. 294–310). Cambridge, UK: Cambridge University Press.

Inglehart, R. (1997). *Modernization and postmodernization*, Princeton: Princeton University Press.

Kurian, G.T. (Ed., 2001). *The illustrated book of world rankings* (5th ed.). Armonk: Sharpe Reference.

LaFromboise, T., Coleman, H., & Gerton, J. (1993). Psychological impact of biculturalism: Evidence and theory. *Psychological Bulletin, 114,* 395–412.

Motti-Stefanidi, F., Berry, J.W., Chryssochoou, X., Sam, D.L., & Phinney, J.S. (in press). Positive immigrant youth in context: Developmental, acculturation and social psychological perspectives. In A. Masten, D. Hernandez & K. Liebkind (Eds.), *Capitalizing on immigration. The potential of immigrant youth.* Cambridge: Cambridge University Press.

Nguyen, A.M.D., & Benet-Martínez, V. (2007). Biculturalism unpacked: Components, measurement, individual differences, and outcomes. Social and Personality Psychology Compass, 1, 101–114

Olweus, D. (1989). Prevalence and incidence in the study of antisocial behaviour: Definition and measurement. In M.W. Klein (Ed.), *Cross-national research in self-reported crime and delinquency* (pp. 187–201). Dordrecht: Kluwer Academic.

Phinney, J.S. (1990). Ethnic identity in adolescents and adults: A review of research *Psychological Bulletin*, 108, 499–514.

Phinney, J.S. (1992). The multigroup ethnic identity measure: A new scale for use with diverse groups. *Journal of Adolescent Research, 7*, 156–176.

Phinney, J., Cantu, C., & Kurtz, D. (1997). Ethnic and American identity as predictors of self-esteem among African-American, Latino and White adolescents. *Journal of Youth and Adolescence, 26*, 165–185.

Phinney, J., & Devich-Navarro, M. (1997). Variations in bicultural identification among African American and Mexican American adolescents. *Journal of Research on Adolescence, 7*, 3–32.

Phinney, J.S., Horenczyk, G., Liebkind, K., & Vedder, P. (2001). Ethnic identity, immigration and wellbeing. An interactional perspective. *Journal of Social Studies,* 57, 493–510.

Portes, P.R. (1999). Social and psychological factors in the academic achievement of children of immigrants: A cultural history puzzle. *American Educational Research Journal, 36*, 489–507.

Portes, A., & Rumbaut, R.G (2006). *Immigrant America: A portrait* (3rd ed.). Berkeley & Los Angeles: University of California

Ryabov, I. (2009). The role of peer social capital in educational assimilation of immigrant youths. *Sociological Inquiry, 79*, 453–480.

Sam, D.L., & Berry, J.W. (2010). Acculturation: when individuals and groups of different cultural backgrounds meet. *Perspectives on Psychological Science, 5*, 472–481

Seligman, M.E.P., Csikszentmihalyi, M. (2000). Positive psychology: An introduction. *American Psychologist, 55*, 5–14.

Sterling, R.W. (1974). *Macropolitics: International relations in a global society.* New York: Knopf.

Suárez-Orozco, C., & Suárez-Orozco, M. (2001). *Children of immigration.* Cambridge: Harvard University Press.

Van de Vijver F.J.R., & Phalet, K. (2004). Assessment in multicultural groups: The role of acculturation. *Applied Psychology: An International Review, 53*, 215–236.

Vedder, P., & Horenczyk, G. (2006). Acculturation and the school. In D.L. Sam & J.W. Berry (Eds.), *The Cambridge handbook of acculturation* (pp. 419–438). Cambridge: Cambridge University Press

Vedder, P., & Van de Vijver, F.J.R. (2006). Methodological aspects: Studying adolescents in 13 countries. In J.W. Berry, J.S. Phinney, D.L. Sam, & P. Vedder (Eds.), *Immigrant youth in cultural transition: Acculturation, identity and adaptation across national contexts* (pp. 47–69). Mahwah: Lawrence Erlbaum Associates.

Vedder, P., Van de Vijver, F.J.R., Liebkind, K. (2006). Predicting immigrant youths' adaptation across countries and ethnocultural groups. In J.W. Berry, J.S. Phinney, D.L. Sam, & P. Vedder (Eds.), *Immigrant youth in cultural transition: Acculturation, identity and adaptation across national contexts* (pp. 167–194). Mahwah, NJ: Lawrence Erlbaum Associates.

Veling, W., Susser, E., van Os, J., Mackenbach, J.P., Selten, J.P., & Hoek, H.W. (2008). Ethnic density of neighborhoods and incidence of psychotic disorders among immigrants. *American Journal of Psychiatry, 165*, 66.

Verkuyten, M. (2005). *The social psychology of ethnic identity.* Hove: Psychology Press.

Verkuyten, M., & Zaremba, K. (2005). Interethnic relations in a changing political context. *Social Psychology Quarterly, 68*, 375–386.

Ward, C. (1996). Acculturation. In D. Landis & R. Bhagat (Eds.), *Handbook of intercultural training* (2nd ed., pp. 124–147). Thousand Oaks: Sage.

Ward, C. (2001). The A, B, Cs of acculturation. In D. Matsumoto (Ed.), *The handbook of culture and psychology* (pp. 411–445). Oxford: Oxford University Press.

David L. Sam
Department of Psychosocial Science, University of Bergen
Christiesgate 12
NO–5015 Bergen (Norway)
Tel. +47 5558 3215, E-Mail david.sam@psysp.uib.no

# Examining Spiritual Capital and Acculturation across Ecological Systems: Developmental Implications for Children and Adolescents in Diverse Immigrant Families

Soojin S. Oh · Hirokazu Yoshikawa

Harvard Graduate School of Education, Cambridge, Mass., USA

## Abstract

Religion and spirituality encompass vibrant and critical contexts for developing children, and have played an integral role in American immigration history. However, a scholarly attention to the role of faiths, spirituality, and religious institutions in the lives of immigrants is a relatively new endeavor. Jasso and colleagues report that Christianity constituted approximately two thirds of the New Immigrant Survey-Pilot immigrants, and over 41% reported attending religious services weekly or more often. Notwithstanding the importance of faith traditions and religious communities to the lives of many immigrant families, spiritual capital has not been applied to understanding the unique experiences and trajectories of immigrant children and youth. This chapter explores the developmental significance of spiritual capital at three levels of social contexts: (1) family settings, (2) social networks, and (3) organizations and institutions. In addition to an interdisciplinary review of the literature, we draw from the MetroBaby Qualitative Studies of the Center for Research on Culture, Development, and Education, to ground our synthesis in longitudinal qualitative data – field notes and parent in-depth interview transcripts drawn from predominantly low-income, Chinese, Dominican and Mexican, first-generation immigrant mothers raising young children. We draw on empirical evidence to theorize how spiritual capital might shape developmental goals and experiences of children of immigrants from infancy to adolescence across proximal settings. To highlight the links between particular settings and specific outcomes, we further identify moderators and developmental mechanisms that add complex layers to our portrayal of spiritual capital in the lives of immigrant families.

Copyright © 2012 S. Karger AG, Basel

Economic and demographic trends have long attested to the importance of immigrants for the American economy. In forthcoming decades, immigrants will be critical for ensuring the welfare of aging baby boomers in the US [Myers, 2007]. The long-term health of American democracy likewise rests on the bedrock of immigrants and their children. In this chapter, we assess how the spiritual capital – religious beliefs, behaviors, practices, and networks – facilitates the production, accumulation, and utilization of other forms of capital among immigrant families. More specifically, we ask how might spiritual and religious attitudes, beliefs, practices, and contexts influence children's daily experiences in immigrant homes? What variations in and possible mechanisms for such effects exist within and across social settings? Through an interdisciplinary review, we synthesize current evidence to illustrate how religious organizations and faith communities operate as critical contexts for shaping immigrant families' daily routines, socialization processes as well as children's ethnic identity development.

While social capital theorists have documented how child development is powerfully shaped by social capital [Coleman, 1988; Putnam, 2000], the developmental significance of spiritual capital has not been applied to investigating the trajectories of immigrant children. In our inquiry of how this important yet understudied dimension of immigrant life shapes child development, we present a conceptual model that highlights multiple dimensions of spiritual capital, predictors of spiritual capital, and links between spiritual capital and various developmental outcomes during childhood and adolescence.

## Demographic and Policy Contexts: Immigration, Religion and Spirituality

Religion and spirituality encompass vibrant and critical contexts for developing children, and have played an integral role in American immigration history – providing institutional resources for social adaptation, personal meaning for interpreting immigration experiences, and continuous force for expanding the national ideal of pluralism [Alba, Raboteau & DeWind, 2008]. Faith-based organizations, in particular, have historically served as key organizations extensively involved in the education and healthcare sectors, with many focused on social inclusion, advocacy, and service provision for newly arriving immigrants in the US and abroad.

Recent national data on newly authorized US immigrants show that approximately two thirds of this group identified themselves as Christian, lower than the 86% of the native-born surveyed in the General Social Survey of 2002. However, the proportion of Catholics among legal immigrants is 42%, almost twice as large as among the native-born, and over 41% reported attending religious services weekly or more [Jasso, Massey, Rosenzweig & Smith, 2005]. Eight percent of the new immigrants identified themselves as Muslim, and 15% reported no religious affiliation.

Immigrants to the US from most parts of the world become more actively involved in faith-based institutions and religious communities after migration than they were in their home countries [Foley & Hoge, 2007]. Scholars have observed increased religious practice and conversion upon arrival among multiple immigrant groups [Smith, 1999; Williams, 1988]. Over 75% of the Korean population in the US is involved with a Christian church, for example, while only 30% profess Christian faith in Korea [Kim & Min, 2002]. Notwithstanding the importance of faith, religious traditions, and spirituality in the lives of many children and adolescents in immigrant families, recent syntheses and overviews of the immigration literature do not document the importance of spirituality or religion at all [Stepick, 2005]. This is a major oversight, given Putnam's [2000] finding that nearly half of all associational memberships, personal philanthropy, and volunteering in the US are faith related [Alba et al., 2008; Iannoccone & Klick, 2003; Ley, 2008].

This chapter explores the developmental significance of spiritual capital at three levels of social contexts: (1) family settings, (2) social networks, and (3) organizations and institutions (fig. 1). In addition to review of relevant literatures, we draw from the MetroBaby Qualitative Studies (MQS) of the Center for Research on Culture, Development, and Education, to ground our synthesis in longitudinal qualitative data – field notes and parent in-depth interview transcripts drawn from predominantly low-income, Chinese, Dominican and Mexican, first-generation immigrant mothers

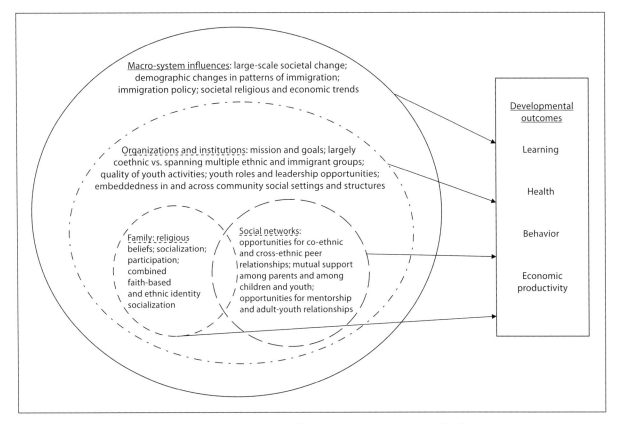

**Fig. 1.** Developmental contexts of spiritual capital for children and youth in immigrant families.

raising young children. This study was conducted in New York City, and aimed to examine the roles of home culture, child care, employment, and policy contexts in shaping development in the first years of life. The qualitative data were collected in a sample of 25 families randomly drawn from a larger sample of 374, with each family visited between 6 and 12 times across child ages 9–30 months (for more details on methods, see Hagelskamp, Hughes, Yoshikawa, and Chaudry [in press] and Yoshikawa [2011]). We draw on both the literature review and this empirical evidence to theorize how spiritual capital might shape developmental goals and experiences of infants and toddlers from immigrant families across proximal settings. To highlight the links between particular settings and specific outcomes, we further identify moderators and developmental mechanisms that add complex layers to our portrayal of spiritual capital in the lives of immigrant families.

**What Is Spiritual Capital?**

Bourdieu [1986] broadly defines capital as accumulated human labor transferred through time in either material or embodied states that can potentially produce different forms of profits for the individual. Capital therefore implies investment strategies and assets both at the individual and group level [Svensen & Svensen, 2003]. Bourdieu's reformulation of Marx's concept of capital suggests that capital exists in both material (physical, economic) and non-material (cultural, symbolic, social) forms. For Bourdieu, one form of capital can be converted into another, and all forms of capital can be converted into economic capital.

We argue that time, energy, and capital investments directly linked to spiritual beliefs and religious participation encapsulate a related yet theoretically different form of capital than what Bourdieu defines as non-material forms of capital. Similarly, assets, membership benefits, relationships, and networks acquired across religious contexts may constitute elements of capital distinct from other social, cultural, and symbolic capital. For instance, Bourdieu's concept of social capital as a form of power facilitates trust and informal exchanges that reduce transaction costs and enhance economic growth. We acknowledge that this definition clearly applies to religious communities and institutions – such organizations have resources linked to group membership, institutionalized relationships of reciprocity, as well as collectively owned financial and other forms of capital. However, the formation of relationships and the nature of these transactions in spiritual communities extend beyond Bourdieu's and Coleman's [1988] understanding of social capital and cannot be limited to their analyses of religious institutions simply as yet another social enterprise [Verter, 2003]. In addition, definitions of spiritual capital offered by others [e.g. Iannoccone, 1990; Stark & Finke, 2000] rest heavily on personal dispositions, which may also be limited. Existing literature either dismisses or underestimates the potential influences spiritual dimensions of interpersonal interactions, social engagement, and life experiences can have on immigrant parents' developmental goals, childrearing practices, family routines, self-identity, and worldviews.

We comprehensively define spiritual capital as characterized by the knowledge, beliefs, behavior, and social networks related to one's religion or spirituality [Iannaccone, 1990; Iannaccone & Klick, 2003; Finke, 2003], with the following characteristics:

- *Multidimensional:* We perceive spiritual capital comprised of multiple dimensions such as religious beliefs, practices, behavior, involvement, participation, knowledge, skills, and networks. We further posit that faith, religiosity, spirituality and religiousness are relevant constructs employed to measure different dimensions of spiritual capital. Such multifaceted conceptualization of spiritual capital can also be understood in terms of its social, cultural, emotional, historical, and intellectual dimensions across diverse religious contexts and social settings.
- *Multi-Leveled:* Spiritual capital operates within and across multiple levels – individual, family, community, and institutional. Though it cannot be separated from the individual [as in human capital; Becker, 1975], it also inheres in the relations among and between members of faith-based communities [as in social capital; Coleman, 1988]. Though spiritual capital does not necessitate formal participation in any level of religious institution, we concentrate our analysis on spiritual capital produced within faith-based organizations due to the limited availability of empirical studies documenting spirituality outside religious communities.
- *Dynamic and Context-Specific:* Multiple dimensions of spiritual capital do not remain static but constantly shift over time. Individuals create and modify spiritual capital based on their evolving understanding of spirituality and religion, and their importance at a particular time in a particular context. Changes and continuities can be observed in spiritual patterns of religious beliefs and behavior over the life cycle, among family and friends, between and across generations [Iannaccone, 1990]. More importantly, spiritual capital operates on a daily, periodic, seasonal, and occasional basis – time scales that are specific to the rhythms, routines and rituals

of communities. In addition, spiritual capital is produced and augmented, diminished and employed across different social settings. Spiritual capital acquired in one context can be transferred to another social setting for further accumulation or utilization [Iannaccone & Klick, 2003; Jaworsky, 2006].

- *Facilitates Economic Productivity:* This idea of spiritual capital-enhancing productivity reflects Weber's [1930] attribution of the emergence of capitalism to Protestantism (e.g. the Protestant work ethic). We posit that spiritual capital can contribute or limit opportunities for creating human, social, economic, and cultural capital that further affect acculturation and integration of immigrants and their children. To the extent that social ties in religious settings facilitate social and economic mobility, spiritual capital may have a link to human, economic and financial capital. Norms tied to religious identities affect economic outcomes [Benjamin, Choi & Fisher, 2010]. To borrow Putnam's [2000] term, spiritual capital 'lubricates' civic society by generating voluntary provisions of collective goods. According to Verter [2003], spiritual capital like other forms of capital similarly consists of 'transforming contingent relations, into relationships that are at once necessary and elective, implying durable obligations subjectively felt' [p. 152]. In this perspective, spiritual capital can also be subject to the laws of accumulation, inheritance, and exchange that govern other forms of capital.

## Predictors of Spiritual Capital

*Individual Dispositions*
Children's developmental characteristics – cognitive, emotional, and personality – can influence the emergence and development of faith. Some early prominent psychologists – William James, and G. Stanley Hall – and many more recent psychologists – Gordon Allport, Carl Jung, Erich Fromm, and Abraham Maslow – have argued that religion or spirituality functions as a core developmental domain and can be seen integrated across the lifespan [Hill et al., 2000]. Closely linked to individual's cognitive functioning, Fowler [1989] points out that spiritual beliefs correlate significantly with one's way of knowing and valuing. Hill and colleagues further describe that a quest orientation to religion may entail complexity of thought, whereas religious fundamentalism may be associated with less complex types of thinking. Religious beliefs may also be conceptualized as schema activated only within believers. On a related note, religious conversion or spiritual experience is tied to personal affect and emotion [Zinnbauer & Pargament, 1998]. Friendship and social networks also create safe spaces for experiencing belonging and interdependence. Human need for belonging and friendship may motivate spiritually inclined children and adolescents to become religiously involved. More debatable is the idea that proposes religion and spirituality as genetic determinants of personality that may predict one's acquisition of spiritual capital. Sociobiological theories emphasize genetic and evolutionary factors that might undergird religious and spiritual beliefs about morality [Wenegrat, 1990; Wilson, 1978]. Additionally, D'Onofrio, Eaves, Murrelle, Maes, and Spilka [1999] posit the heritability of religious behaviors and attitudes.

*Family History and Practice of Religion and Spirituality*
Families critically shape the spiritual development and religious experiences of children and youth in multiple ways. The religious roots of a family and multigenerational spiritual lineages can have powerful influences on children's exposure to certain doctrines and their early participation in particular religious rituals and communities. The intertwinement of collective history and religious upbringing shared amongst family members, within a child's most immediate and personal setting, may influence his or her

religious beliefs and behaviors over a course of a lifetime. More than two thirds of the adults who attended a Korean church as children still belong in a Korean American congregation [Min & Kim, 2005]. The presence of grandparents and relatives can reinforce the centrality of religious faith and spiritual life in multiple ways. These adults help children to make meaning out of major life events, learn codes of conduct, and engage in moral reasoning. Some of this family socialization may involve negotiating mainstream rituals in the host country. One Dominican mother in the MQS, for example, explained to the fieldworker her reason for not allowing her son to go trick or treating on Halloween:

> As I stood outside of Lorena's (grandma's) apartment, I heard the grandma saying goodbye to Alberto (the focus child, 14 months) and telling him 'dile adios a mama' ('say goodbye to mama'). Lorena takes care of the baby most of the time and seems to make decisions about how he should be raised. Claudia [Alberto's mother] explained that he was not going trick or treating because Lorena was a Christian and did not want Alberto to be part of Halloween that she saw as a pagan festivity.

Young children are also exposed to adults' discussion about death, funeral rites, afterlife, and religious propriety as another Dominican family observes the Holy Week in anticipation of Easter:

> The person whom Nuris [mother] took care of had died and she had been trying to reach the family to give her condolences. While she was on that call, Nuris's parents, her aunt, and her uncle stopped by to say hi on their way to church for Holy Thursday. They talked about the woman's death and about the funeral. The woman had asked to be cremated and Altagracia started saying that, as a Catholic, she was against that and that the church condemned that. They also talked about the Holy Week's religious activities and Altagracia started to lecture the kids on how they had not gone to any of the religious activities that week. They looked at her with a shameful smile and told her that they would go to mass on Sunday.

Likewise, one adolescent participant, Diego, from Pearce and Denton's [2011] study articulates how his family has influenced his faith:

> My ideas about God come from my parents. Um, that's where they all originated[d]. Before my grandma passed away, she was a big influence. She was very religious. She kind of taught me how to pray – the right way to pray. And she was the one that really pushed, you know, the whole religion thing. And, being Catholic is something my parents taught me through church [p. 57].

Some immigrant families intricately integrate ethnic socialization of their children and religious education as articulated by Delgado-Bernal [1998] – a Mexican scholar who highlights how her family's socioeconomic background, history, and Catholic religious ideology simultaneously shape her epistemological lens. Her account further exemplifies how multigenerational family members may support a child to acquire spiritual capital as an intellectual asset in later years. She argues that through the experiences of ancestors and elders, Chicanas and Chicanos impart knowledge of conquest, loss of land, social segregation and resistance, and labor market. Delgado-Bernal [1998] recollects, 'As a child, my own family experience included learning through my grandmothers' stories, which were sprinkled with religion and mysticism, and my father's stories about the urban challenges of his childhood' [p. 303].

*Macrosystemic Forces*

Dynamic systems theory suggests that influences of spiritual capital on child and youth development can occur across ecological levels, in directions from macro to micro, micro to macro, or even skipping levels [Yoshikawa & Hsueh, 2001]. For example, policy edicts by major religious denominations could affect child and youth development through intervening community or family mechanisms. Consider the acceptance of ordination of women ministers, priests, imams or rabbis in particular denominations of Christianity, Islam, or Judaism. Such a policy shift would be widely publicized within the religious communities, and family conversations about the shifts would influence girls' and boy's conceptions of sex roles and what it means to be a leader in a religious community. Such influences might also occur through parents' socialization and messages about the policy, conveyed intentionally or unintentionally to children.

Large-scale economic change can drive the particular religious demographic that predominates in particular waves of migration. Economic factors have largely driven waves of low-income migration from Latin America and China to the US [Yoshikawa, 2011], with consequences for religious membership and participation. For example, large recent Mexican waves of migration have increased the numbers of Catholics in the US, and driven the growth of some denominations (e.g. Pentecostal congregations). In some cases, congregations and denominations have grown as a result of ties to immigrant communities (e.g. the Chinese church). These patterns ultimately affect the development of the second generation, who participate alongside their parents in their early years, and often into adolescence.

Since religion and spirituality are inherently social-psychological phenomena, Hill et al. [2000] theorize that reference groups and cultural norms are rooted in religious perspectives, prescribing an acceptable range of alternatives for normative behavior. For instance, regardless of the level of religiosity or spirituality, most individuals living in the Southern states along the Bible Belt tend to be socioculturally Christian, immigrants and native-borns alike. On a different note, religious persecution experienced by immigrant families prior to migration might affect whether and how they would develop spiritual beliefs or engage in religious practices. In fact, some immigrant families have fled their land in pursuit of religious freedom in the US. On the other hand, immigrant families whose coethnics in contexts of reception have established a wide network for religious organizations providing access to services, resources, and community may feel more incentivized to become religiously involved than they had been in their home country. Using the New Immigrant Survey-Pilot data set, Cadge and Ecklund [2006] systematically considered, for the first time, how demographic, familial, employment, household language, and migration factors influence regular religious service attendance amongst new immigrants from different religious traditions. They argue that immigrants who are less integrated into various facets of American society are more likely to attend religious services regularly, lending further support to how immigrants' ties to their ethnic communities influence their religious participation. Our analysis corroborates this phenomenon: among three immigrant groups – Mexicans, Dominicans, and Chinese – the Mexicans, the group with the highest proportion undocumented and reporting the lowest levels of overall social support availability, reported the highest levels of church attendance [Yoshikawa, 2011].

## Spiritual Capital across Developmental Periods

What does the development of religious beliefs and involvement look like across childhood, as children progress from more biologically determined participation in fewer contexts to environmentally and self-driven choice of contexts in adolescence [McCall, 1981]. Fowler [1981, 1989] proposes stages of faith, closely related to Kohlberg's moral development stages. During infancy to age 2, this stage 0 or the 'Primal Faith', is characterized by the development of trust and forming bonds of attachment to primary caregivers, largely shaped by consistency and responsivity of caregivers [Erikson, 1963; Fowler, 1981, 1989]. The 'Intuitive-Projective Faith', or stage 1 applies to children from toddlerhood to early childhood. During this critical period of brain development, young children develop their gross motor, fine motor, and cognitive skills. Piaget's preoperational stage also emerges during this period as the child engages in symbolic representational play. During this phase, young children initially begin benefitting from parents' acquisition and eventual accumulation of spiritual capital and usually follow the beliefs of their parents. Some parents influence their children's religious or spiritual development through verbal communication and indoctrination of beliefs, disciplinary norms, and behavioral modeling [Roehlkepartain, Benson, King & Wagener, 2006]. For example, one of the Dominican mothers in the MQS study has taught her 14-month-old daughter the importance of bedtime prayer. The infant learned early on to adopt the religious behavior of their parents as described below:

> Martha reinforces Sophie's behavior as she adds that Sophie has also learned how to pray her night prayer before she goes to bed. Then Martha starts to say a prayer of 'a guardian angel' and Sophie places her hand in front of her chest and follows up with Martha completing the last words of each sentence that Martha says, mumbling the rest of the prayer. We are both smiling back at Sophie as she acknowledges a sense of approval and smiles back at us. Then she continues to play with the wooden pieces of her animal's puzzle. Since attending mass is part of the family routine, Sophie has learned to say, 'misa mami' (mommy mass), when she hears Martha getting ready to go to the church.

Fowler's stage 2, 'Mythical-Literal Faith', occurs during early and middle childhood, when beliefs in fairness and justice, goodness and reciprocity emerge during children's play and may be linked to religious or spiritual beliefs and experiences. Children of this period also create anthropomorphic representations of deities and respond to religious stories and rituals in literal, not symbolic, ways. According to Fowler [1989], young children's spiritual aptitude coupled with spiritual nurturance, discipline, and practice provided by families and religious communities may lead some children to a deeper and more rapid development of spirituality. Many immigrant children spend the majority of their time in extended family networks, primarily with their grandparents [Suarez-Orozco, Suarez-Orozco & Todorova, 2008]. Within this family structure more common to the daily experiences of immigrant children, first-generation grandparents can play an influential role in cultivating their grandchildren's spiritual development while reinforcing religious attitudes and behavior.

Although parents play an important role on religious discipline and spiritual experience of their children initially, adolescents become central agents in choosing to continue their adherence and participation in religious institutions. The positive youth development framework [Lerner, Roeser & Phelphs, 2008] has explicitly identified spirituality and religiosity as individual and community-level assets that promote positive developmental features such as healthy identity formation, civic engagement, and purpose [Dowling et al., 2004]. Much recent scholarly attention has focused on the role of spirituality and religiosity on adolescents since this particular period for some adolescents signifies important changes and growth in spiritual and religious domains [Good & Willoughby, 2008]. Religious and spiritual beliefs and practices may change, along with the biological, psychological and social transitions in adolescence: puberty, increased autonomy and independence, sexual interest, self-discovery, identity development, and a concern for the future [Pearce & Denton, 2011]. Adolescents also experience key life transitions such as driving, working, voting, attending college, parenting – each context may influence how adolescents choose to and become religiously active or not during their youth and into their adulthood. With more freedom to determine their own behaviors, adolescents may also follow guidelines from their faiths in making difficult decisions. They might also reject their own family religiosity as they try to establish autonomy and adhere to more North American youth values.

Religion plays a significant role in many adolescents' lives [Pearce & Denton, 2011; Smith & Denton, 2005]. Contrary to dominant perceptions, Pearce and Denton [2011] present evidence that youth in the US surveyed since 2002 have remained or have gotten more religious during their teenage years. Data from the Gallup Youth Survey indicate that adolescents are more religious – in their attitudes, beliefs, and behavior – during their early teen years, with church or synagogue attendance declining near entry into adulthood [Gallup International Institute, 1999]. In comparison to adolescent boys, adolescent girls report higher levels of religiousness [Donahue & Benson, 1995], religious judgment [Oser & Gmunder, 1991], positive religious coping, and daily spiritual experiences [DesRosiers & Miller, 2007]. For adolescents from non-religious homes, attending college geographically far from home may provide new opportunities to explore spirituality by joining campus-based religious groups where some end up forming positive and negative social relations, reciprocate information and resources, and experience spiritual support from peers and mentors.

Most teenagers follow the religious beliefs and practices of their parents, becoming involved with the religious congregations in which they were raised and professing religion to be an important part of their lives [Pearce & Denton, 2011; Smith & Denton, 2005]. Despite the prominence of religion as reported by adolescents, Smith and Denton explain that religion remains an often unfocused and implicit aspect of their lives: Most adolescents have difficulty articulating the meaning, influence, and implications of their beliefs for themselves and the world. Fowler [1981, 1989] would frame one such experiences in his stage 3, 'Synthetic-Conventional Faith', during which adolescents' experience of the world extends beyond family and faith, may provide a coherent orientation and synthesize values to provide a basis for their emerging identity. Fowler further argues that this stage for many adults becomes a permanent place of equilibrium – a conformist stage that tunes to external expectations and judgments while grappling to construct one's autonomous perspective.

Unlike theoretical presentations of developmental stages as proposed by Kohlberg and Fowler, Pearce and Denton [2011] developed an alternative conceptualization of faith amongst adolescents in the US by presenting five unique profiles of youth religiosity. Their large study explores the religious and spiritual dimensions of middle adolescents by analyzing the first and second waves of the National Study of Youth and Religion telephone surveys amongst youth aged 13–17 in 2002, and conducted in-depth interviews with more than 120 youth aged 16–21 at two time points. By comparatively exploring the nonreligious characteristics of youth in relation to these religious profiles in their study, Pearce and Denton came to understand how adolescents become religious. The five unique profiles of religiosity – Abiders, Adapters, Assenters, Avoiders, and Atheists – conceptually represent adolescents' different approaches to religion. Predictors of these religious expressions are personal temperament and individual agency, socioeconomic factors, ethnic and gender identity, and family religious background that collectively shape adolescents' spiritual inclinations and pull them in particular directions. Adapters comprised of 20% of the sample who expressed strong belief in and connection to a personal God believed that religion is inspirational to them, but were not the most regularly involved in churches, temples, or mosques, either by choice or circumstances. Avoiders represented 24% of the sample; these youth profess some belief in God but engage in rare or no religious practice. The authors found no significant difference in self-reported measure of happiness and health between Atheists and other profiles. However, Atheists smoke, drink alcohol, and engage in sexual activity significantly more than other youth [Pearce & Denton, 2011].

Based on these findings, authors argue that it is not simply the presence or absence of religion in one child's life that leads to happiness and health but rather, a well-articulated system of belief and meaning regardless of religious affiliation. However, these belief systems – religious or not – are heavily informed and constructed through adolescents' interactions with their parents. Particularly for immigrant parents who may experience linguistic barriers with their American-born children or have long working hours away from home, these parents may feel limited to fully support their second-generation children to internalize and systematically articulate spiritual beliefs as their own. The question remains as to what extent these five profiles proposed by Pearce and Denton reflect the diverse approaches to religious faiths and spiritual trajectories largely affected by immigrant family life.

The development of spiritual capital among immigrant youth involves intersectionality of ethnic identity, gender, cultural adjustment, and nativity status. Almost half of first-generation immigrant students in one large study reported that most of their friends share their ethnic and immigrant backgrounds [Suarez-Orozco et al., 2008]. According to Suarez-Orozco and colleagues, forming companionship with peers from the same country of origin appears to be particularly important for newly arrived children and youth because they support one another to become acclimated to a new school, a new neighborhood, or a new city. These students find that coethnic immigrant peers in youth groups are often organized by ethnic worship communities. Friendships formed within these religious spaces, forged by shared faith and immigration experience, further allow the more experienced students to serve as important informants on school culture, US education system, citizenship, and mainstream culture. Furthermore, immigrant peers may experience safety by belonging in ethnic religious organizations where their formative experiences, observations of parental struggles, family hardships, and language barriers affirm their social realities.

**Spiritual Capital in Family Settings**

Religious beliefs and socialization reside most centrally within families, as influences on child and youth development in immigrant families.

*Family Religious Beliefs*
The role of religious and spiritual beliefs in family life in child development begins at birth. The conception and birth of a child carry important spiritual meaning commonly portrayed by major religions as a divine miracle or a blessing from God [Mahoney, Pargament, Murray-Swank & Murray-Swank, 2003]. Families in religious communities celebrate the spiritual significance of birth and early life of their child in the presence of these communities (e.g. Catholic Christening ceremonies, Protestant infant baptisms, Jewish circumcisions, Aqeeqah – Islamic birth ritual, or Hindu naming ceremonies). Religious communities further promote rites of passage that signify important developmental transitions such as Catholic Communion, and the Jewish Bar Mitzvah or Catholic Confirmation, when early adolescents publicly profess their faiths and moral responsibility.

In our study, almost all (16 out of 18) the Mexican and Dominican families described the importance of Catholic faith and the significance of planning for the infant baptism. Because baptism celebrations require time and resources, some families mentioned that they planned to have enough saved to afford a baptism ceremony when their babies turn 2 years old. In most cases, the baptism service was held in Spanish at a nearby neighborhood Catholic Church, followed by a small party where relatives and close friends were invited. In other occasions, families saved up to have infant baptisms in Mexico in order to involve a larger family network.

I: Would you want for the girls to visit Mexico?
M: Yes, we want to go, but I tell you, just for that, to baptize them over there with the entire family.

Below, we provide an illustrative excerpt from the field notes that describe the infant baptism that integrates religious tradition, family gatherings, and ethnic cultural practices:

We finally got to Miguel's birthday party. There were a lot of friends and family there and of all ages: babies, teenagers, their parents, and older people. They had balloons, birthday ornaments, and a big cake with the Winnie the Pooh ornament that Miguel had pointed at before. The music in the background was mostly reggaeton, bachata, and merengue. Everyone was dancing to it, including Miguel, who was dancing with another baby girl. . . There was a woman, a family's friend, who said a prayer for Miguel and his family. She focused on health and family unity and at the end poured holy water on Miguel's head. They also lit a candle and everyone said the Lord's Prayer.

While parents may welcome parenting as a divine gift or an answered prayer [Mahoney et al., 2003], studies find mixed results regarding the influence of parent religious beliefs on children. On the one hand, Brody and Flor [1998] found in their African-American sample that greater maternal religiosity is significantly associated with more 'no nonsense' parenting, harmonious mother-child relationships, and educational involvement. Mahoney et al. [2003] found that mothers who reported higher levels of spiritual meaning in parenting, on average, used less verbal aggression with their children aged 4–6. In contrast, Bottoms, Shaver, Goodman and Qin [1995] attest to religious motivations for child abuse and neglect. Through their examination of religion-related child abuse cases, authors confirm cases involving parents' withholding of medical care for religious reasons, or abuse perpetrated by religious authority figures. Furthermore, children and youth who experience cognitive dissonance between the actual reality and the ideals of family relationships as professed by their religious traditions may experience exacerbated relational maladjustment, guilt, anger, and helplessness [Mahoney et al., 2003].

*Family Spiritual and Religious Socialization*
The socialization of children and youth in spiritual and religious matters is an underexamined aspect of parenting and family socialization in immigrant families. Yet from the standpoint of the intergenerational transmission of spiritual capital, this is perhaps a primary pathway for intergenerational continuity or discontinuity in spiritual capital. To take one example of socialization, religious and spiritual traditions expose children to norms about relationships, commitment, and marriage. For example, Protestantism proclaims that marital relationship between a man and a woman is reflective of the covenantal love between the Christ and the Church. We observed that several Mexican and Dominican immigrant mothers were taking Confirmation classes so that they can be married by the Church. Similar to infant Baptism, an official acknowledgement of marriage by the Catholic Church appears to be important for these parents and would potentially shape how their children perceive the role of religious membership on marriage and family. Within Judaism, the relationships among family members are reflective of the covenant between God and the people of Israel. We speculate that religious beliefs and traditions may influence how children and adolescents view romance, marriage, and family thereby informing their worldviews and interpersonal relations. Multiple studies support that family religious participation is positively associated with children's marital patterns later as indicated by greater levels of marriage, lower marital infidelity, less domestic violence, and lower divorce probability [Benjamin et al., 2010; Burdette, Ellison, Sherkat & Gore, 2007; Ellison, Trinitapoli, Anderson & Johnson, 2007; Gruber, 2005].

Many parents' desire to incorporate religion as part of their children's lives draws them back into faith communities but might have stronger significance for immigrant families. Immigrant parents may also reinforce the ethnic identity development of their children by expanding exposure to cultural norms, traditions, and practice inherent in immigrant ethnic faith communities. Further, we note that facilitating children's identification with ethnic cultural attitudes reinforced in these religious communities tends to be easier for families with newly arrived immigrant children than for immigrant households with US-born children. The following example illustrates how religious socialization can serve the function of retaining the culture of the country of origin.

After describing different important Catholic religious days celebrated in Mexico – the Day of the Dead, the Day of the Virgen de Guadalupe, and the Day of the Semana Santa (Easter) – this mother from our study expressed her desire to instill the significance of these religious cultural traditions for her 1-year-old daughter.

> For her not to ignore that, I mean, for her to know what that [religious tradition] signifies and to know how to show respect during those holidays. And not because she is far away to forget about them, or not to feel Mexican because she is from here... I plan on start talking to her about that, so that she will never forget. Yes, because, if I don't explain anything to her, then she will never know anything. It's just like the people from here, they don't value that. The religion is over there [Mexico], the cultures, all that, it doesn't signify anything for all those who moved over here! They know about it, but it doesn't have any value for them. And that is not what I want to happen to her.

Another Mexican mother spoke about how she teaches her children cultural and religious lessons about the Virgin of Guadalupe as a Mexican cultural symbol. The young boy then associates his mother's motherland, Mexico, and family religious traditions. The desire to return to a homeland that he has never known is accentuated by the Mexican tradition of the Virgin of Guadalupe.

> I tell my children, 'Oh, she is the Virgin of Guadalupe of the Basilica in Mexico.' Then my children tell me, 'and where is that?' and I tell them, 'in Mexico.' And they ask, 'and how, how?' I mean, they ask me about how the Virgin came to be. 'The Virgin appeared in Mexico, there in the villa, there is where she appeared, and from there she went to all the countries.' 'How did she do that?' [Laughs] they ask me. So I say, 'well, she went everywhere, and anywhere she can and there she stays forever. I tell him 'Do you want to go to Mexico?' And he says, 'Yes, when I grow up I'm going to go.' He says, 'I'm going to go where you said the Virgin appeared.'

In accordance with this ethnographic evidence, family religious participation appears related to developmental outcomes in large-scale studies. In examining the Early Childhood Longitudinal Study consisting of over 9,000 kindergarteners and first graders, Bartowski, Xu and Levin [2008] argue that parent religiosity is positively associated with a range of child psychological and social adjustment outcomes in early childhood such as social competence, lower incidence of internalizing and externalizing behavior problems, and more advanced cognitive ability. Using data from the National Survey of Families and Households, Wilcox [2001] indicates that residential fathers who report being involved in a religious organization are more likely to have dinner with their children, get involved in youth-related activities (e.g. Boy Scouts, local sports leagues), and this effect is particularly significant amongst low-income families. Analyses of 3,124 low-income fathers from the Fragile Families and Child Wellbeing Study reveal that the birth of a child is associated with an increase in fathers' religious participation, and further, their religious participation is significantly associated with positive father engagement even after controlling for religious affiliation, marital status, relationship transition, pro-fathering attitudes, and first-time fatherhood [Petts, 2007]. More interestingly, first-time fathers with high levels of religious participation also report the highest father engagement with their children in early childhood [Petts, 2007; Roggman, Boyce, Cook & Cook, 2002].

However, religious socialization can also exclude certain groups of children and youth growing up in religious families, such as LGBT or gender-nonconforming youth. In part for religious reasons, families can reject gay youth, with severe consequences for their well-being and health. For example, family rejection among gay Latino youth growing up in immigrant families is related to higher rates of depression, suicidality, drug use, and unprotected sex [Ryan, Huebner, Diaz & Sanchez, 2008]. Latino gay men report hearing consistent family messages growing up about the shame that homosexuality brings on the family [Sandfort, Melendez & Diaz, 2007]. In response to these influences, religious organizations specific to LGBT communities have arisen within Christian and Jewish traditions to integrate spiritual capital with LGBT identity, which can be marginalized in mainstream religious institutions [Brettschneider, 2006; Rodriguez & Ouellette, 2002]. In some instances, religion supports the exclusion for the family for youth's following non-approved self-chosen, life course decisions, such as dressing (body exposure, tattoo, body piercing), cohabitation, marrying members of other religions.

## Spiritual Capital across Social Networks

*Ethnic Social Networks, Fictive Kinship and Peer Influences*
Religious traditions and faith are often shared by most, if not all, of the immediate family members, and can help introduce children in immigrant families to larger social networks of ethnic community members. Immigrant parents use spiritual capital to create social opportunities for children and youth to engage and interact with peers, mentors, and other adults in immigrant worship communities. This can occur for both adults and mentor figures outside the family, as well as peers. In their description of ethnic variations in fictive kinship systems among newly arrived immigrants, Ebaugh and Chafetz [2000] explain that *Compadrazgo* is a complex system of coparenthood commonly practiced among Latino immigrants. Compadrazgo exists throughout Latin America, and intricately interweaves Catholic custom and ritual requiring spiritual sponsorship at baptism. This baptismal compadrazgo system ensures that the primary sponsor or the godparent(s) fulfills both the spiritual and social obligations by providing for the material welfare and instructing the child on faith and morals, in the event that parents die or neglect their spiritual duty. The compadrazgo network extends beyond the triadic relationship between the baptized child, biological parents, and godparents when different sponsors are selected for the first communion, confirmation, and marriage, thus increasing the number of support network members who are committed to the child across his or her entire development.

One Mexican mother of an 8-month-old infant explained her reasons for choosing their roommate, Adam, as her son's godfather:

The godfather is like 'another dad'. If we ever need help or support with Eduardo, Adam will help however he can. Since he is unmarried, we could not make his wife a godmother. We did not choose my sister-in-law as a godmother since she is already supportive and helpful with Eduardo. Baptism would not make her any more helpful or give Eduardo any more support because she offers it readily. Since Adam has become a trusted friend of the family, I feel that making Adam the godfather would encourage him to continue or increase support for Eduardo.

Some of the specific benefits for children and youth of multiple godparent figures may include the presence of multiple adult figures modeling spiritual disciplines, availability of emotional support, and provision of material resources. Similarly, Suarez-Orozco et al. [2008] indicate that 'child fostering', a widely accepted cultural practice in the Caribbean, occurs frequently during migration when families in hardship temporarily entrust their children to extended relatives back 'home'.

The developmental implications of parent networks may vary depending on the presence or absence of children during these network gatherings. One example of institutionally based immigrant parent networks for young children is illustrated in Jaworsky's [2006] study. To describe how spiritual capital transfers beyond religious contexts, Jaworsky examined a group of Brazilian immigrant parents spiritually driven to 'use their gifts not only for their immediate family but for others' who formed a long-lasting parent network for young children. In building and strengthening organizational ties across various government agencies and faith-based institutions, a representative leader attested, 'We have groups that have been working on early childhood now since the middle '90s, arm in arm with like 10 or 15 agencies, that we're almost like one... There is a sort of vertical and horizontal integration in how we're working together...' [p. 25]. These parent leadership programs empower parents to learn information on available programs and services, and acquire resources that they can share with other immigrant parents in their communities.

Peer networks of children and youth themselves are a second important dimension of spiritual capital at the social network level on children and youth. Children's time spent with their peers grows over time as their independence from parents might increase. Roehlkepartain et al. [2006] argue that deep sensitivity and connection with friends provide a transcendent experience that may provide the foundation for the spiritual development of children and adolescents. For example, friends have added unique variance over and above that of parental influence in adolescents' experience of the divine and the importance of religion. Schwartz [2006] found that adolescent religious belief and involvement can be explained by engaging in conversations about faith with their peers and being exposed to their friends' faith modeling. Religious participation can give them access to peers that do not engage in risky behaviors.

Religious network exposure may restrict certain kinds of peer characteristics. To the extent that faith-based networks are primarily coethnic, for example, opportunities to meet and interact with peers of different ethnicities and backgrounds may be restricted. Most faith-based networks are restricted to a single faith, and therefore exposure to peers of different faiths may also be limited. The potential for conflict between contexts with different levels of diversity in faith and therefore peer characteristics – e.g. public schools vs. coethnic, faith-based social networks – exists and has been reported in the youth development literature.

**Spiritual Capital in Organizations and Institutions**

*Immigrant Worship Community Characteristics*
Immigrant worship communities provide unique developing contexts for cultivating immigrant children's cultural attitudes and ethnic identification. Religious beliefs and practices play an integral part of ethnic identity in many immigrant communities and constitute an important mechanism for ensuring cultural continuity in the second generation [Ebaugh & Chafetz, 2000]. Most often, we find that ethnic socialization and religious practices are intertwined across many social settings in which immigrant families interact with their child(ren). Immigrant faith communities preserve important cultural facets by combining cultural traditions and religious rituals to support ethnic identity development of children growing up in these immigrant communities.

Immigrant worship communities promote ethnically bounded socialization goals as well as cultural models that can be contested and adapted by their children and adolescents. More specifically, immigrant children and adolescents actively engaged in their faith communities acquire necessary language, tools, and norms to navigate competing social and religious contexts – developing culturally bounded spiritual capital while converting cognitive and social assets that may predict children's engagement and learning in school. Many second-generation children growing up in Chinese and Korean immigrant families participate in Saturday language schools that also offer classes on ethnic history, cultural celebrations, arts, dance, and sports [Kim & Min, 2002; Min & Kim, 2005]. Recent studies have found positive effects of heritage language proficiency and usage on adolescents' social and mental health outcomes. Heritage language was positively associated with the quality of parent-adolescent relationships and ethnic identity, suggesting that the development of proficiency in the heritage language facilitates successful cultural adjustment among first- and second-generation Asian and Latino adolescents [Oh & Fuligni, 2010]. Additionally, non-English home language use was found to be the only setting-level variable, predicting above and beyond all peer-related characteristics, as a protective factor for first-generation Latino and Asian adolescent risk behavior [Garcia-Coll et al., 2011]. These findings suggest that home language maintenance provides many psychological and social benefits for immigrant adolescents. Immigrant worship communities that provide heritage language programs provide additional opportunities for children and adolescents to practice the language of their immigrant parents and broaden access to participate in their parents' primary culture and ethnic communities, thereby contributing to a strong sense of ethnic identity and connection to cultural traditions.

*Private Religious Schools*

Religious private schools can facilitate academic engagement as well as spiritual development of immigrant students who might otherwise feel marginalized in schools where they do not have the opportunities to interact with coethnic peers or other students of immigrant background. First, religious doctrine powerfully undergirds the institutional mission, school culture, and pedagogical approaches to learning across disciplines. School policy on admission, student conduct and discipline, parent involvement, bullying and conflict resolution largely reflect religious values promoted across home and school. Religious schools similar to faith-based organizations reinforce family norms and routines around spiritual and religious socialization. Such consistency in moral expectations and codified rules across social settings may support adaptation of newly arriving immigrant students.

Dominican immigrant parents in our study spoke of their preference for Catholic schools over public education. Some parents were spending a significant portion of family income to afford tuition costs for elder siblings of the focus child. Consistent alignment of behavior norms, expectations, and standards across home and school might also support children's acculturation process. Second, religious teachings can also shape the nature and quality of student-teacher interactions as well as peer relationships in school context. Particularly for immigrant students who are experiencing family separation, emotional support from teachers as mentor figures who share their faith traditions and life outlook can increase their relational engagement in school [Suarez-Orozco et al., 2008].

More interestingly, immigrant faith communities are actively employing social capital formed within religious spaces to facilitate the formation of spiritual capital for their children. Emerging communities of immigrant parents and religious leaders are joining the charter schools movement in many states to create a learning space that differs greatly from most public schools for their children. Basford [2010] describes how a key group of Muslim immigrant parents and educators collectively envisioned an alternative schooling space for their 1.5 generation East African Muslim high school students who simultaneously navigate racial, ethnic, linguistic, geographic, and religious labels in their acculturation process. Facilitation of spiritual capital among a Somali school board and East African-born teachers allowed for an education institution that promotes holistic development of students who experience multiple forms of marginalization. The school's explicit focus on nurturing religious identity permeated across all aspects of the school climate where 'Islam is not seen simply as a religion to practice. Rather, to nearly all of my participants, being a Muslim is a way of life, and often how they primarily identify themselves' [p. 11]. Basford [2010] further notes that such phenomenon is part of a larger and important trend in the charter school movement where more than 30 out of 138 charter schools in Minnesota are ethnocentric in orientation. These counterspaces represent an immigrant religious community's collective resistance to preserve rich ethnic, cultural, and religious aspects of their life and empower their children to seamlessly integrate their religious life and spiritual disciplines across contexts. These immigrant school communities extend the original contribution of Coleman's [1988] seminal study that illustrates the importance of constructing schooling spaces where students are not forced to subtract certain parts of their identity, but to come as their fullest selves – including their religious beliefs. The Catholic schools in Coleman's study served as a construction site for bonding social capital amongst parents, teachers, school administrators, and neighbors to positively influence their students' academic outcomes. African Islamic charter school in Basford's study and Catholic schools in Coleman's both exemplify how students in these school communities benefited from possessing greater social capital formed through a network closure among family, friends, and non-relative adults who also know one another, encounter on a regular basis, and share similar values.

*Children and Adolescents in Faith-Based Organizations*

Faith-based organizations may provide cognitively enriching environments for immigrant children to acquire knowledge and develop academic skills in relation to their religious doctrine, which, in turn, can be converted into other forms of capital in different social settings. Based on parent-reported measures of child religiosity, children who engage in religious activities perform significantly better on a range of cognitive and socioemotional outcomes than children who do not [Dye, 2008]. Also, Marietta [2010] presents a case study of an Appalachian county in Eastern Kentucky where churches play a central role in developing language and literacy amongst low-income children. Regardless of religious beliefs and affiliation, she asserts that church played a nearly inescapable role in children's lives through exposure to oral messages and texts including 'prayers being said before lunch at Pizza Hut, religious signs placed along mountain roads, or Bible stories being shared at school' [p. 12] as well as exposure to sophisticated literacy experiences and academic vocabulary. While Gruber [2005] points out that increased religious participation among youth is associated with later higher educational attainment and less use of social welfare programs, Parke and Buriel [2006] note that religious involvement in 8th grade is predictive of academic and social competence by the 12th grade. Additionally, faith-based organizations offer other supplementary services or low-cost extracurricular programs for immigrant children to attend afterschool or during the summer. Some Vietnamese Catholic and Protestant congregations provide formal ethnic programs, weekend religious training, and summer camps for second-generation children. Moreover, Easton-Waller [2000] further reports that monks from Cambodian Buddhist temples provide mentoring guidance for youth members; these programs and services are positively associated with high educational attainment [Bankston & Zhou, 1996].

Developmental effects of spiritual capital extend beyond cognitive and educational outcomes. Moreover, studies report that spirituality and religiosity of adolescents aged 13–19 year olds are associated with their sympathy and perspective taking [King & Furrow, 2004] and prosocial behavior amongst youth in grades 6–9 [Benson, Scales, Sesma & Roehlkeptartain, 2006]. Studies further demonstrate how youth involvement in faith-based activities may serve as protective factors against behavioral risks. Youth religious participation is associated with lower substance use and heavy drinking for both parents and youth, negatively related to suicide ideation and attempts, premature sexual involvement as well as smoking, drinking, criminal and delinquent behavior [Ball, Armistead & Austin, 2003; Dehejia, DeLeire, Luttmer & Mitchell, 2007; Donahue & Benson, 1995; Gruber & Hungerman, 2006; Johnson, De Li, Larson & McCullough, 2000; Johnson, Jang, Larson & De Li, 2000; Pearce, Jones, Schwab-Stone & Ruchkin, 2003]. However, the magnitude of the relation between religiosity with risk behaviors such as aggression and delinquency appears to be very modest [Good & Willoughby, 2008; Johnson et al., 2000].

Although religious beliefs and participation in immigrant families show positive effects on children's identity and other aspects of development, this may not always be true. There is some evidence that for mental health, in particular, associations with religious participation can be just as likely to be positive as well as negative. In some studies, for example, higher rates of participation are linked to higher levels of stress (e.g. higher frequency of prayer [Ellison, Boardman, Williams & Jackson, 2001]). This may be due to the well-known association of social support provision with higher stress. Seeking spiritual support and benevolent religious appraisals were associated with better mental health, while other kinds of coping, such as appraisal of gods or deities as punishing, were associated with worse mental health [Pargament, Tarakeshwar, Ellison & Wulff, 2001].

Associations of immigrant worship community involvement with youth outcomes are not always positive. One study found, for example, that perceived social support from adolescents' religious community was associated with lower levels of depressive symptoms; however, perceived criticism and demands from their religious organization were associated with higher levels of depressive symptoms [Pearce, Little & Perez, 2003]. Although religious organizations provide spaces for recreational activities and promote prosocial behavior (e.g. community service, cooperation, empathy, and altruism), they can also in some cases be associated with youth gang activities [Parke & Buriel, 2006]. This can be especially true in the context of unstructured and unsupervised youth activities, a characteristic of youth programs that is generally associated with higher antisocial behavior [National Research Council, 2002]. Activities within a program can differ in their associations with youth outcomes, based on adult/youth ratios, focus of the program and other characteristics [Shinn & Yoshikawa, 2008]. For youth in immigrant families, ethnicity-specific schooling such as Chinese shadow schooling programs, many of which have some religious affiliation, can intensify academic pressure in the lives of some youth [Zhou, 2008]. Finally, Dew, Daniel, Goldston and Koenig [2008] confirm that depression among outpatients aged 12–18 was positively related to negative religious experiences.

Furthermore, spiritual meanings and religious significance defined and reinforced by many organized institutions may privilege those children growing up in families whose experiences fit the traditionally prescribed sacred family structure (e.g. heterosexual marriage), while marginalizing children whose family structure and functioning remain outside the norm as defined by many religious communities (e.g. single-parent households, blended families, children of gay couples). Deloria [1994] impugns how one faction of the Christian community dangerously harms their children. The Jesus movement operated by a charismatic summer camp in North Dakota is infamously noted to have caused psychic injury on young children and youth who were brainwashed to adopt fanatic ideas that further lead to bigotry, intolerance, and distorted perceptions of social realities.

Another negative influence of religion can be seen in Hunsberger's [1995] investigation of the relationships among right-wing authoritarianism, religious fundamentalism, and prejudice towards racial minority groups. Even after controlling for educational background, he finds that college students who scored high on the Right-Wing Authoritarianism scale, on average, also scored significantly high on the Religious Fundamentalism scale, racial prejudice, and the Attitudes toward Homosexuals Scale that reflects condemning and vindictive sentiments towards LGBT individuals. Some adults who align with fundamental religious denominations and profess conservative religious or moral values believe LGBT students – actual or perceived – do not deserve protection and support [Poteat, 2008; Swearer & Cary, 2003]. While religious participation may provide a clear sense of purpose and identity, fundamentalist views can severely narrow children's definition of morality and negatively affect their perception of others who hold differing views or life choices. Also, young women in many religions encounter conflicting tensions in adolescence when autonomy and deindividuation are more prevalent as gender-related norms and expectations espoused by religious traditions clash with postmodern views regarding femininity and womanhood.

**The Study of Spiritual Capital among Immigrant Families: Implications for Research, Practice and Policy**

The spiritual and religious life of immigrant communities has rarely been linked to the development of children and youth in those communities. This chapter has aimed to present an ecological model for how spiritual capital may matter for immigrant families. As the US is transformed by the influx of new communities in recent decades, the concomitant transformation of spiritual and religious life has been overlooked. We have described in this chapter a multidimensional model of spiritual capital, encompassing beliefs, practices, and behaviors. In addition, our model has incorporated multiple ecological and dynamic levels of analysis, from the individual to family, peer, organizational, institutional and large-scale demographic and policy contexts. All of these must be considered in a comprehensive model of how spiritual capital can impact children and youth in immigrant families.

The study of immigration and immigrant families can contribute substantially to the literature on religion and spirituality among children and youth. The diversity of practices and organizations, and the relationship between involvement in countries of origin and contexts of reception in the US, can enrich the study of youth involvement in religions. The diversity of youth beliefs and practices among immigrant groups, for example, has rarely been considered in either local or national studies of religious participation. The religious and spiritual experiences of immigrant children and youth, in addition, are inextricable from organizational and neighborhood contexts of reception, and as such bring much-needed foci on influences beyond the individual and family to the broader developmental literature on religiosity.

Conversely, the study of spiritual capital can enrich the literature on immigrant children and youth. Processes of segmented assimilation and acculturation have rarely been studied as they play out in the family and organizational socialization of first, second- and third-generation immigrant youth. For instance, what effect does spiritual capital have on the individual child's selective assimilation and selective preservation of ethnicity in the process of negotiating multiple identities? The protective processes associated with religious involvement in youth, for example, may be an important and overlooked component of the well-known protective effect of retention of one's heritage and ethnic identity among the second generation [Portes & Rumbaut, 2001]. Isolating immigrants from mainstream institutions – by self-selection or not – may increase prejudice toward the other groups and limit social opportunities for young people to engage others from diverse backgrounds. Coethnic religious organizations constitute a large and visible portion of the influence of ethnic enclaves on youth – this specific part of the enclave story, similarly, has been missing from the literature on immigrant child development (except by sociologist Portes, Rumabut and others). Finally, the potential of religious organizations to foster incorporation on other dimensions – political, economic, and social – has been overlooked. In recent ethnographies, faith-based organizations have shown the potential to reach new immigrant communities, providing opportunities for empowerment and advocacy, not just spiritual and social support [Catone, Chung & Oh, 2011; Galvez, 2009; Yoshikawa, 2011; Zlolniski, 2006]. In large part, this is because these organizations have gained the trust of immigrant communities in a way that traditional social service organizations, businesses and even schools cannot, even in coethnic contexts.

Research on spiritual capital and its effects on immigrant youth is nascent and requires attention to several dimensions. First and most fundamentally, general studies of child and youth development in immigrant families should as a rule explore the religious and spiritual aspects of these families' lives. The major studies of immigration and youth development, for example, have only glanced at this important context of immigrant communities and development. This is an enormous gap in our understanding of the contexts of children's development in immigrant families. Second, examining the longitudinal trajectories of spiritual capital, across developmental periods and across immigrant generations, is vital in order to delineate how spiritual capital enriches processes of acculturation, positive youth development, and ultimately inter-generational mobility among immigrant families. Third, mediators and moderators of the association of spiritual capital with positive outcomes have not been explored for immigrant youth. For whom do positive associations hold most strongly, and for whom are they less positive or even negative? How exactly does religious participation produce positive effects on particular domains of development?

Finally, research on spiritual capital and its development in immigrant families has the potential to inform practice and policy related to immigration. Immigrant worship communities provide unique sites for newly arriving immigrants to acquire spiritual capital that, in turn, can be converted to other forms of capital not readily accessible to them in the mainstream society. First, the practices of faith-based organizations in immigrant communities that enhance youth development could be documented much more extensively, with principles drawn out for the work of community-based organizations. As organizations that immigrant families trust, these settings may incorporate important practices for the development of social capital that could be applied to those serving other types of families, or other types of organizations serving newcomer communities. Second, the role of these organizations in building developmentally responsive immigration policies has been underestimated. Networks of congregations, for example, can serve as effective venues for advocacy and community organizing for 'hard-to-reach' newcomer groups, some of which are among the most disadvantaged in the nation [Warren & Mapp, 2011; Yoshikawa, 2011]. Finally, the development of leaders in communities cutting across spiritual, political, and economic dimensions is urgent for immigrant groups. Combating institutional discrimination and racism toward immigrant groups, such as the recent wave of violence against Latina/o communities, for example, requires leadership from multiple kinds of organizations, including faith-based ones. As leaders and communities work together across boundaries defined by race, ethnicity, socioeconomic status, political power, and religion, newcomers across the nation can develop a more powerful and effective voice to broaden pathways for future generations, contributing to strengthening and revitalizing the fabric of American civic life.

## References

Alba, R., Raboteau, A.J., & DeWind, J. (2008). *Immigration and religion in America*. New York: New York University Press.

Ball, J., Armistead, L., & Austin, B.J. (2003). The relationship between religiosity and adjustment among African-American, female, urban adolescents. *Journal of Adolescence, 26*, 431–446.

Bankston, C.L., & Zhou, M. (1996). The ethnic church, ethnic identification, and the social adjustment of Vietnamese adolescents. *Review of Religious Research, 38*, 18–37.

Bartowski, J.P., Xu, X., & Levin, M.L. (2008). Religion and child development: evidence from the early childhood longitudinal study. *Social Science Research, 37*, 18–36.

Basford, L. (2010). From mainstream to East African charter: Cultural and religious experiences of Somali youth in U.S. schools. *Journal of School Choice: Research, Theory, and Reform, 4*, 485–509.

Becker, G.S. (1975). *Human capital: A theoretical and empirical analysis, with special reference to education.* Cambridge: National Bureau of Economic Research.

Benjamin, D.J., Choi, J.J., & Fisher, G.W. (2010). *Religious identity and economic behavior.* (NBER Working Paper No. 15925). Cambridge: National Bureau of Economic Research.

Benson, P.L., Scales, P.C., Sesma, A., & Roehlkepartain, E.C. (2006). Adolescent spirituality. *Adolescent and Family Health, 4*, 41–51.

Bottoms, B.L., Shaver, P.R., Goodman, G.S., & Qin, J. (1995). In the name of God: A profile of religion-related child abuse. *Journal of Social Issues, 51*, 85–111.

Bourdieu, P. (1986). Forms of capital. In Richardson, J.G. (Ed.), *Handbook of theory and research for the sociology of education.* (pp. 241–258). New York: Greenwood Press.

Brettschneider, M. (2006). *The family flamboyant: Race politics, queer families, Jewish lives.* Albany: SUNY Press.

Brody, G.H., & Flor, D.L. (1998). Maternal resources, parenting practices, and child competence in rural, single-parent African American families. *Child Development, 69*, 803–816.

Burdette, A., Ellison, C., Sherkat, D., & Gore, K. (2007). Are there religious variations in marital infidelity? *Journal of Family Issues, 28*, 15–53.

Cadge, W., & Ecklund, E.H. (2006). Religious service attendance among immigrants: Evidence from the new immigrant survey-pilot. *American Behavioral Scientist, 49*, 1574–1595.

Catone, K., Chung, C.K., & Oh, S.S. (2011). An appetite for change: Building relational cultures for educational reform and civic engagement in Los Angeles. In M. Warren & K.L. Mapp, (Eds.), *A match on dry grass: Community organizing as a catalyst for school reform.* London: Oxford University Press.

Coleman, J.S. (1988). Social capital in the creation of human capital. *American Journal of Sociology, 94*(supplement), S95–S120.

Dehejia, R., DeLeire, T., Luttmer, E.F.P., & Mitchelle, J. (2007). *The role of religious and social organizations in the lives of disadvantaged youth.* (NBER Working Paper No. 13369). Cambridge: National Bureau of Economic Research.

Delgado-Bernal, D. (1998). Using a Chicana feminist epistemology in educational research. *Harvard Educational Review, 68*, 555–582.

Deloria, R. (1994). *God is red: A native view of religion.* Golden: Fulcrum Publishing.

DesRosiers, A., & Miller, L. (2007). Relational spirituality and depression in adolescent girls. *Journal of Clinical Psychology, 63*, 1021–1037.

Dew, R.E., Daniel, S.S., Goldston, D.B., & Koenig, H.G. (2008). Religion, spirituality, and depression in adolescent psychiatric outpatients. *The Journal of Nervous and Mental Disorders, 196*, 247–251.

Donahue, M.J., & Benson, P.L. (1995). Religion and the well-being of adolescents. *Journal of Social Issues, 51*, 145–160.

D'Onofrio, B.M., Eaves, L.J., Murrelle, L., Maes, H.H., & Spilka, B. (1999). Understanding biological and social influences on religious attitudes and behaviors: A behavior-genetic perspective. *Journal of Personality, 67*, 953–984.

Dowling, E.M., Gestsdottir, S., Anderson, P.M., von Eye, A., Almerigi, J., & Lerner, R.M. (2004). Structural relations among spirituality, religiosity, and thriving in adolescence. *Applied Developmental Science, 8*, 7–16.

Dye, J. (2008, July). *Children's religious attendance and child well-being: 2004.* Paper presented at the annual meeting of the American Sociological Association, Boston, MA.

Easton-Waller, B. (2000). Mean street monks. *Tricycle, 10*, 60–66.

Ebaugh, H.R., & Chafetz, J.S. (2000). *Religion and the new immigrants: Continuities and adaptations in immigrant congregations.* New York: AltaMira Press.

Ellison, C.G., Boardman, J.D., Williams, D.R., & Jackson, J.S. (2001). Religious involvement, stress, and mental health: Findings from the 1995 Detroit area study. *Social Forces, 80*, 215–249.

Ellison, C., Trinitapoli, J., Anderson, K., & Johnson, B. (2007). Race/ethnicity, religious involvement, and domestic violence. *Violence Against Women, 13*, 1094.

Erikson, E.H. (1963). *Childhood and society.* (2nd ed.). New York: Norton.

Finke, R. (2003). Spiritual capital: Definitions, applications, and new frontiers. Prepared for the Spiritual Capital Planning Meeting, October 10–11.

Foley, M.W., & Hoge, D.R. (2007). *Religion and the new immigrants: How faith communities form our newest citizens.* New York: Oxford University Press.

Fowler, J.W. (1981). *Stages of faith: The psychology of human development and the quest for meaning.* San Francisco: HarperSanFrancisco.

Fowler, J.W. (1989). Strength for the journey: Early childhood development in selfhood and faith. In D. Blazer (Ed.), *Early childhood and the development of faith* (pp. 1–36). Kansas City, MO: Sheed and Ward.

Gallup International Institute (1999). *The spiritual life of young americans: Approaching the year 2,000.* Princeton: Author.

Galvez, A. (2009). *Guadalupe in New York: Devotion and the struggle for citizenship rights among Mexican immigrants.* New York: New York University Press.

Garcia-Coll, C., et al. (2011, April). Documenting and explaining the behavioral immigrant paradox in adolescence: The roles of individual and context characteristics. Paper presented at the 2011 Society for Research in Child Development Biannual Meeting, Montreal.

Good, M., & Willoughby, T. (2008). Adolescence as a sensitive period for spiritual development. *Child Development Perspectives, 2*, 32–37.

Gruber, J. (2005). Religious market structure, religious participation, and outcomes: Is religion good for you? *Advances in Economic Analysis and Policy, 5*, 1–30.

Gruber, J., & Hungerman, D.M. (2006). *The church vs. the mall: What happens when religion faces increased secular competition?* (NBER Working Paper No. 12410). Cambridge, MA: National Bureau of Economic Research.

Hagelskamp, C., Hughes, D., Yoshikawa, H., & Chaudry, A. (in press). Negotiating motherhood and work: A typology of role identity associations among low-income, urban women. *Community, Work and Family.*

Hill, P.C., Pargament, K.I., Hood, R.W., McCullough, M.E., Swyers, J.P., Larson, D.B., & Zinnbauer, B.J. (2000). Conceptualizing religion and spirituality: Points of commonality, points of departure. *Journal for the Theory of Social Behavior, 30,* 51–77.

Hunsberger, B. (1995). Religion and prejudice: The role and religious fundamentalism, quest, and right-wing authoritarianism. *Journal of Social Issues, 51,* 113–129.

Iannaccone, L.R. (1990). Religious practice: A human capital approach. *Journal for the Scientific Study of Religion, 29,* 297–314.

Iannaccone, L.R., & Klick, J. (2003, October). Spiritual capital: An introduction and literature review. Prepared for the Spiritual Capital Planning Meeting, Cambridge, MA.

Jasso, G., Massey, D.S., Rosenzweig, M.R., & Smith, J.P. (2005). The New Immigrant Survey Pilot (NIS-P) Public Release Data. Retrieved from http://nis.princeton.edu.

Jaworsky, N. (2006, October). The medium and the message: The form and content of socio-spiritual capital in a new American gateway. Prepared for presentation at the 5th annual conference of the Association for the Study of Religion, Economics, and Culture (ASREC), Portland, OR.

Johnson, B.R., De Li, S., Larson, D.B., & McCullough, M. (2000). A systematic review of the religiosity and delinquency literature. *Journal of Contemporary Criminal Justice, 16,* 32–52.

Johnson, B.R., Jang, S.J., Larson, D.B., & De Li, S. (2000). Does adolescent religious commitment matter? A reexamination of the effects of religiosity on delinquency. *Journal of Research in Crime and Delinquency, 38,* 22–44.

Kim, J.H., & Min, P.G. (Eds.) (2002). *Religions in Asian America: Building faith communities. (Critical perspectives on Asian Pacific Americans).* Walnut Creek: AltaMira Press.

King, P.E., & Furrow, J.L. (2004). Religion as a resource for positive youth development: Religion, social capital, and moral outcomes. *Developmental Psychology, 40,* 703–713.

Lerner, R.M., Roeser, R.W., & Phelphs, E. (2008). *Positive youth development and spirituality: From theory to research.* West Conshohocken, PA: Templeton Foundation Press.

Ley, D. (2008). The immigrant church as an urban service hub. *Urban Studies, 45,* 2057–2074.

Mahoney, A., Pargament, K.I., Murray-Swank, A., & Murray-Swank, N. (2003). Religion and the sanctification of family relationships. *Review of Religious Studies, 44,* 220–236.

Marietta, S.H. (2010). The role of church in promoting literacy in a rural, low-income community. Paper presented at the 42nd annual New England Education Research Organization conference. Unpublished manuscript: Harvard Graduate School of Education.

McCall, R. (1981). Nature-nurture and the two realms of development: A proposed integration with respect to mental development. *Child Development, 52,* 1–12.

Min, P.G., & Kim, J.H. (2005). Intergenerational transmission of religion and culture: Korean Protestants in the U.S. *Sociology of Religion, 66,* 263–282.

Myers, D. (2007). *Immigrants and boomers: Forging a new social contract for the future of America.* New York: Russell Sage.

National Research Council and Institute of Medicine, Committee on Community-Level Programs for Youth. (2002). *Community programs to promote youth development.* Washington, DC: National Academy Press.

Oh, J., & Fuligni, A.J. (2010). The role of heritage language development in the adjustment of adolescents from immigrant backgrounds. *Social Development, 19,* 202–220.

Oser, F., & Gmunder, P. (1991). *Religious judgment: A developmental perspective.* Birmingham: Religious Education Press.

Pargament, K.I., Tarakeshwar, N., Ellison, C.G., & Wulff, K.M. (2001). Religious coping among the religious: The relationships between religious coping and well-being among a national sample of Presbyterian clergy, elders, and members. *Journal for the Scientific Study of Religion, 40,* 439–513.

Parke, R.D., & Buriel, R. (2006). Socialization in the family: Ethnic and ecological perspectives. In W. Damon, & R.M. Lerner (Eds.) *Handbook of child psychology: Social, emotional, and personality development. Vol. 3: Social, Emotional, and Personality Development Chapter 8* (6th ed., pp. 429–501). Hoboken: John Wiley & Sons.

Pearce, L., & Denton, M.L. (2011). *A faith of their own: Stability and change in the religiosity of America's adolescents.* New York: Oxford University Press.

Pearce, M.J., Jones, S.M., Schwab-Stone, M.E., & Ruchkin, V. (2003). The protective effects of religiousness and parent involvement on the development of conduct problems among youth exposed to violence. *Child Development, 74,* 1682–1696.

Pearce M.J., Little T.D., & Perez J.E. (2003). Religiousness and depressive symptoms among adolescents. *Journal of Clinical Child Adolescent Psychology, 32,* 267–276.

Petts, R.J. (2007). Religious participation, religious affiliation, and engagement with children among fathers experiencing the birth of a new child. *Journal of Family Issues, 28,* 1139–1161.

Portes, A., & Rumbaut, R.G. (2001). *Legacies: The story of the immigrant second generation.* Los Angeles and Berkeley, CA: University of California Press.

Poteat, V. (2008). Contextual and moderating effects of the peer group climate on use of homophobic epithets. *School Psychology Review, 37,* 188–201.

Putnam, R.D. (2000). *Bowling alone: The collapse and revival of American community.* New York: Simon & Schuster.

Rodriguez, E.M., & Ouellette, S. (2002). Gay and lesbian Christians: Homosexual and religious identity integration in the members and participants of a gay-positive church. *Journal for the Scientific Study of Religion, 39,* 333–347.

Roehlkepartain, E.C., Benson, P.L., King, P.E., & Wagener, L.M. (2006). Spiritual development in childhood and adolescence: Moving to the scientific mainstream. In E.C. Roehlkepartain, P.E. King, L. Wagener & P.L. Benson (Eds.) *The handbook of spiritual development in childhood and adolescence* (pp. 1–15). Thousand Oaks, CA: Sage.

Roggman, L.A., Boyce, L.K., Cook, G.A., & Cook, J. (2002). Getting dads involved: Predictors of father involvement in Early Head Start and with their children. *Infant Mental Health Journal, 23,* 62–78.

Ryan, C., Huebner, D., Diaz, R.M., & Sanchez, J. (2008). Family rejection as a predictor of negative health outcomes in White and Latino lesbian, gay and bisexual young adults. *Pediatrics, 123,* 346–352.

Sandfort, T.G.M., Melendez, R.M., & Diaz, R.M. (2007). Gender nonconformity, homophobia, and mental distress among Latino gay and bisexual men. *Journal of Sex Research, 44,* 181–189.

Schwartz, K.D. (2006). Transformations in parent and friend faith support predicting adolescents' religious faith. *The International Journal for the Psychology of Religion, 16,* 311–326.

Shinn, M., & Yoshikawa, H. (Eds.) (2008). *Towards positive youth development: Transforming schools and community programs.* New York: Oxford University Press

Smith, J.I. (1999). *Islam in America.* New York: Columbia University Press.

Smith, C., & Denton, M.L. (2005). *Soul searching: The religious and spiritual lives of American teenagers.* New York: Oxford University Press.

Stark, R., & Finke, R. (2000). *Acts of faith: Explaining the human side of religion.* Berkeley, CA: University of California Press.

Stepick, A. (2005). God is apparently not dead: The obvious, the emergent, and the still unknown in immigration and religion. In K.I. Leonard, A. Stepick, M.A. Vasquez, & J. Holdaway, J. (Eds.), *Immigrant faiths: Transforming religious life in America.* (pp. 11–38). Walnut Creek, CA: AltaMira Press.

Suarez-Orozco, C., Suarez-Orozco, M., & Todorova, I. (2008). *Learning a new land: Immigrant students in American society.* Cambridge, MA: Harvard University Press.

Svenson, G.L., & Svenson, G. (2003). On the wealth of nations: Bourdieuconomics and social capital. *Theory and Society, 32,* 607–631.

Swearer, S., & Cary, P. (2003). Perceptions and attitudes toward bullying in middle school youth: A developmental examination across the bully/victim, continuum. *Journal of Applied School Psychology, 19,* 63–79.

Verter, B. (2003). Spiritual capital: Theorizing religion with Bourdieu against Bourdieu. *Sociological Theory, 21,* 50–174.

Warren, M., & Mapp, K.L. (Eds.) (2011). *A match on dry grass: Community organizing as a catalyst for school reform.* London: Oxford University Press.

Weber, M. (1930). *The Protestant ethic and the spirit of capitalism.* New York: HarperCollins (original text first published 1905).

Wenegrat, B. (1990). *The divine archetype: The sociobiology and psychology of religion.* Levington, MA: Lexington Books.

Wilcox, W.B. (2001). *Good dads: Religion, civic engagement, & paternal involvement in low-income communities.* Philadelphia: Center for Research on Religion and Urban Civil Society.

Williams, R.B. (1988). *Religions of immigrants from India and Pakistan: New threads in the American tapestry.* New York: Cambridge University Press.

Wilson, E.O. (1978). *On human nature.* Cambridge, MA: Harvard University Press.

Yoshikawa, H. (2011). *Immigrants raising citizens: Undocumented parents and their young children.* New York: Russell Sage.

Yoshikawa, H., & Hsueh, J. (2001). Child development and public policy: Toward a dynamic systems perspective. *Child Development, 72,* 1887–1903.

Zhou, M. (2008). The ethnic system of supplementary education: Nonprofit and for-profit institutions in Los Angeles' Chinese immigrant community. In M. Shinn & H. Yoshikawa (Eds.), *Toward positive youth development: Transforming schools and community programs* (pp. 229–253). New York: Oxford University Press.

Zinnbauer, B.J., & Pargament, K.I. (1998). Spiritual conversation: A study of religious change among college students. *Journal for the Scientific Study of Religion, 37,* 161–180.

Zlolniski, C. (2006). Janitors, street vendors, and activists: The lives of Mexican immigrants in Silicon Valley. Berkeley, CA: University of California Press.

Soojin Susan Oh
49 Leslie Road
Belmont, MA 02478 (USA)
E-Mail soojinsoh@gmail.com

# Immigrant Youth and Discrimination

Paul Vedder · Mitch van Geel

Department of Education and Child Studies, Leiden University, Leiden, The Netherlands

## Abstract

Many immigrants face some form of discrimination at some point in their lives. This experience may have severe consequences for immigrants' well-being. Our specific focus is on discrimination in schools, and what schools may do to create positive interethnic relations, thus minimizing discrimination. Our choice to focus on schools is firstly inspired by the notion that they serve children and adolescents, age groups that may be affected more severely by discrimination, as they lack the cognitive and emotional capacities to deal with such experiences. Secondly, the classroom may be the most likely place for intensifying and improving the quality of interethnic contact, hence for avoiding or combating discrimination, but also a setting were discrimination is likely to be encountered, from classmates and even from teachers and other significant adults. First, we review the effects discrimination may have on victims. We then shift our attention to the school context to find out how discrimination takes shape through and in schools. We continue with a review of research on what can be done by the victims to protect themselves or by others to protect the victims. We further specify what can be done to (a) improve student's coping capacities and (b) create harmonious interethnic relations in the classroom. Using new data, we argue that a positive school climate is related to fewer experiences of discrimination among students. As such, schools and teachers are able to take important steps to reduce negative intercultural experiences.

Copyright © 2012 S. Karger AG, Basel

Migration is a universal phenomenon, driven mostly by the hopes for a better life. Migration may not only improve the lives of immigrants, it also may help to solve shortages of both lowly and highly skilled laborers in industrialized countries [Lowell & Gerova, 2004]. Despite difficulties, many immigrants enjoy good physical, behavioral and psychological health, sometimes even better than that of their national peers [Garcia Coll & Marks, 2009, in press]. Although many immigrants do well, some face a path of downward assimilation [Portes & Zhou, 1993], and as such it should not be assumed that immigration always leads to positive outcomes. Contexts of exit and reception and other acculturation experiences have important effects on the outcomes of the migration process.

This chapter focuses on the role of discrimination, an aspect of the receiving context, and a factor that might lead to more negative outcomes of the acculturation process in the new immigrants. Many immigrants face some form of discrimination at some point in their lives [e.g. Berry,

Phinney, Sam & Vedder, 2006a], and as will be argued further on in this chapter, the experience of discrimination may have severe consequences for immigrants' well-being. Our specific focus will be on discrimination in schools, and what schools may do to create positive interethnic relations, thus minimizing discrimination. Our choice to focus on schools is firstly inspired by the notion that they serve children and adolescents, age groups that may be affected more severely by discrimination, as they lack the cognitive and emotional capacities to deal with such experiences [Van Geel & Vedder, 2009]. Secondly, the classroom may be the most likely place for intensifying and improving the quality of interethnic contact, hence for avoiding or combating discrimination [Masson & Verkuyten, 1993], but also a setting where discrimination is likely to be encountered, from classmates and even from teachers and other significant adults [Rosenbloom & Way, 2004].

First, we will review the effects discrimination may have on victims. We then shift our attention to the school context to find out how discrimination takes shape through and in schools. After this, we continue with a review of research on what can be done by the victims to protect themselves or by others to protect the victims. We further specify the general notions on individual coping strategies to analyze in the school context what can be done to (a) improve student's coping capacities and (b) create harmonious interethnic relations in the classroom. The latter will be further clarified by presenting new data that will demonstrate what schools may do to reduce discrimination and its negative effects on students.

## Discrimination and Its Effect on Health

Discrimination may have many adverse effects on health. Empirical studies support the notion that negative relations exist between the experience of discrimination and physical and psychological health. The difference in hypertension rates between African-Americans and white Americans has been argued to be due to the persistent discrimination African-Americans endure. To a certain extent, empirical data support this notion as immigrants and minorities that report more experiences of discrimination also report more cardiovascular conditions [Harris et al., 2006], diabetes [Karlsen & Nazroo, 2002], respiratory disease and heart disease [Gee, Spencer, Chen & Takeuchi, 2007] and black women who report experiencing more discrimination give birth to babies with low birth-weight more frequently [Mustillo et al., 2004]. Experiments indicate that experiences of discrimination raise blood pressure [e.g., McNeilly et al., 1995; Merritt, Benett, Williams, Edwards & Soller, 2006], and these rises in blood pressure may eventually translate into a range of poor health outcomes [e.g. Psaty et al., 2001].

However, an alternative explanation for these findings is that the relation between discrimination and physical health is mediated by unhealthy behaviors. It has been found that people that report more experiences of discrimination report smoking more cigarettes [Bennett, Wolin, Robinson, Fowler & Edwards, 2005] and drinking more alcohol [Yen, Ragland, Greiner & Fisher, 1999]. The higher substance abuse among those who are frequently discriminated may, at least partly, explain their comparatively poor physical health. Regardless of the reasons, the adverse effects that the experience of discrimination may have on health should be recognized, even if it is mediated by unhealthy behavioral practices.

In addition, there is a growing literature of the effects of racism on youth. Pachter and Garcia Coll [2009] review the studies of racism and health in youth samples. They conclude that racism is negatively related to mental health and behavioral outcomes in children. Furthermore, racism was found related to increased tobacco and alcohol use, a similar finding as that with adults described above. However, there are fewer studies on the relations between racism and physical health in youth, and as such Pachter and Garcia Coll [2009] argue that more studies on racist experiences in youth samples are needed.

Although the effects of discrimination on health are substantial, a systematic review by Paradies [2006] reveals that the consequences of discrimination for victims' psychological health are at least as grave. People that frequently experience discrimination are found to experience a lower self-esteem [Verkuyten, 1998], a higher level of depression [cf. Noh & Kaspar, 2003; Finch, Kolody & Vega, 2000; Brown et al., 2000], more stress [cf. Sellers, Caldwell, Schmeelk-Cone & Zimmerman, 2003; Brown et al., 2000], higher levels of somatization and anxiety [Bowen-Reid & Harell, 2002], and less positive psychological well-being in general [Berry et al., 2006a; Jasinskaja-Lahti & Liebkind, 2001; Liebkind, Jasinskaja-Lahti & Solheim, 2004]. Those who report high levels of discrimination are also found to engage in violent behaviors more often [Caldwell, Kohn-Wood, Schmeelk-Cone, Chavous & Zimmerman, 2004].

Experiences of discrimination may also contribute to attitudes among youth that are detrimental for their positive development. For example Portes and Zhou [1993], and Ogbu and Simons [1998] describe the existence of subversive youth cultures. The immigrant and minority youth belonging to these youth cultures, existing mainly of coethnic peers, feel that the society they live in is so discriminatory and unfair that they will not receive a fair chance, no matter how hard they work. They come to define working on an education as a 'white thing' or 'selling out', and instead develop behavior that is disruptive or even criminal. Evidence so far comes from small qualitative studies. The regularities observed clearly await further support in large quantitative studies. Hitherto, the rejection identification model [Branscombe, Schmitt & Harvey, 1999] provides some support for these notions. It was found that as a reaction to discrimination, people will choose to define themselves more strongly as a member of their own group, instead of as a member of a national majority that discriminates them. Youth may be particularly vulnerable, lacking coping skills and in turning away from the national majority, may end up in a detrimental youth culture. However, in a study by Marks et al. [2007] concerning children in immigrant families, it was found that, though for some, ingroup identification is indeed related to fewer outgroup friends, among other children from immigrant backgrounds, a stronger ingroup identification coincided with more outgroup friends. The rejection identification model clarifies that the experience of discrimination may lead to ingroup identification and outgroup rejection, but to understand all the mechanisms of ethnic identity, the use of more encompassing models is necessary [e.g. Phinney, Horenczyk, Liebkind & Vedder, 2001; Vedder & Phinney, in press].

Clearly, the existence of discrimination is no small matter, given the many negative consequences it may have. Fortunately however, discrimination may be combated, and the effects of discrimination on health may be alleviated or even nullified. Clark and Gochett [2006] for example found that personal coping may reduce the effects discrimination has on blood pressure. The work of Krieger and Sydney [1996] suggests that African-Americans that challenge unfair treatment experience less of the negative impact of discrimination on blood pressure than those who accept unfair treatment, and in their review Van Geel and Vedder [2009] point out that social support may be of great help when dealing with experiences of discrimination. Especially the work on physical health has been conducted with adults, so there is a need of replication and extending these findings to children and youth.

## The Role of Discrimination in Schooling

Some researchers attribute the outcomes of children from immigrant and minority backgrounds to a variety of factors, avoiding an attribution to discrimination. Stevens [2007] and Stevens, Clycq, Timmerman and Van Houtte [2011] analyzed research on race and ethnicity related educational inequality in Great Britain and the Netherlands, respectively. In both countries, research shows considerable differences between ethnic groups' academic performance, but in both countries researchers also shed doubt on whether these differences can be explained by or interpreted in terms of discrimination. In both countries, most research focuses on school outcomes and in one way or another tries to explain these differences by differences in resources available to students and their families. They do not directly measure discrimination or perceived discrimination. Instead, they refer to differences in socioeconomic status (SES), in educational resources, and differences in proficiency in the language of instruction. They point at a suboptimal fit between student competencies and requirements for learning defined by school, teachers and curriculum developers. That schools are better places for high SES children and children that are more proficient in the language of instruction and that some parents can afford to pay fees for schools with better resources are circumstances that are taken for granted by these researchers. They seem to be inspired by a rather common and broadly used definition of discrimination: making unjustified negative attributions to persons or groups in particular task situations. Unjustified is further defined in terms of personal or group characteristics that are irrelevant to the task accomplishment in the particular situation [e.g. Equal Opportunity Commission of the Government of South Australia, 2010]. They show that SES, language proficiency, and all the other attributes mentioned before do impact on learning performance. Based on their own research, they conclude that these attributes are relevant to the task situation and hence, using those attributes is not discriminatory. By using this 'twist' they suggest that if at all there is someone to blame it is the children's parents who did teach their children the wrong values, language, and did not cater for adequate resources that would allow their offspring to level the achievements of the better off, Caucasian or European children [Garcia Coll et al., 1996].

Other researchers, but also policy makers, teachers and parents may consider this research, the outcomes and interpretations, as expressions of institutional discrimination. To counter it, they may try to define and create instructional and learning situations that are likely to be conducive to the development of lower SES children or whose L1 differs from the language of instruction. They may want to create adaptive cultural settings or contexts within the existing schools' structures. These are settings or contexts that are characterized by accepting, defining and transmitting goals, values, attitudes and behavior characteristic of a particular cultural or ethnic group, and that set the group apart from the dominant culture. It is a way to shelter from or to cope with negative social stratification. Moreover, it is expected that these settings lead to the development of competencies that are not standard or nationally common, but that allow minority children to navigate their lives in a variety of cultural contexts, supportive as well as aversive ones [cf. Garcia Coll et al., 1996].

Although the type of reasoning represented by Stevens et al. [2011] is still quite common, educational research on discrimination in the meantime has resulted in the development, qualification and proliferation of alternative theoretical models. A first one deals with low teacher expectations of children who are seen as members of particular minority groups and a second is the identity model of schooling [cf. Foster, 2008]. The model of *low teacher expectation* contends that low expectations of children's capabilities to learn and achieve are linked to particular ethnic groups. As a consequence, this model can also be described as referring to teacher stereotypes. Groups that are targeted are Afro-Caribbean mainly in European countries and in the USA, African-American kids who are depicted as having limited learning capacities, not willing to be docile and prone to aggression [Mac an Ghaill, 1989; Tenenbaum & Ruck, 2007], Latino kids who are seen as lacking parental support to do well in school, including girls who do not want to violate traditional sex roles [Zentella, 2005] and Asian kids who are depicted as model minorities, social conformists and hard working [Lee, 1994]. These expectations or stereotypes seem to have consequences for interactions between teachers and students, and these interactions may lead to or contribute to the fulfillment of the teachers' expectations.

The second model is Akerlof and Kranton's *identity model of schooling* [2002] which suggests that persons belonging to a minority group, who strongly identify with that group, also adapt to or follow the norms, rules or behavioral prescriptions characteristic of the group in terms of particular measures of adaptation. In the case of groups with low levels of academic aspirations, this may lead to low academic performance. Kromhout and Vedder [1996] showed that for Afro-Caribbean children, particularly boys, this meant that they tended to be more outgoing, disturbing in social settings or slightly more aggressive than other children. This behavior in this group was shown to be reinforced within their own peer group and even maintained by Afro-Caribbean youth immigrated to the Netherlands, although the Dutch peers definitely did not approve of it. This suggests that these behavioral characteristics are normative for these groups, and they identified with the minority identity. The identity model of schooling is inspired by Ogbu's model [Ogbu & Simons, 1998] of oppositional culture that postulates that particular minority groups (involuntary minorities) define norms, rules, and develop behavioral prescriptions that are explicitly oppositional to common notions of the majority group or to particular practices characteristic of the majority culture. This particular substantiation of the identity model of schooling is used more in American (US) than European studies [Heath, Rothon & Kilpi, 2008; Kromhout & Vedder, 1996].

Apart from these models which specifically address teacher-student or school-student relationships, a more common stress-coping model seems to apply in studies showing that students are harassed by classmates because of their ethnic background [e.g. Verkuyten & Thijs, 2002]. This may impair students' academic performance and well-being. However, whether this happens depends on students' coping strategies. As shown by Modood [2004], Asian students in Britain experience more harassment than Afro-Caribbean students, but the Asian students' academic performance does not suffer. Modood attributes this to the different coping strategies used.

As pointed out earlier, most research on discrimination in schools has problems with conceptualizing discrimination. Garcia Coll et al. [1996] argue that researchers too easily contend that behavioral and performance differences between ethnic groups are not caused by discriminatory educational structures and practices. Instead, they try to find alternative explanations that eventually blame the students themselves, their parents or wider social and educational environment. The earlier mentioned stress-coping model in a sense circumvented these problems by focusing on perceived or experienced discrimination. Instead of looking for an objective measure of discrimination, researchers working with stress-coping models started asking persons to indicate the extent or intensity of discrimination experiences [Noh & Kaspar, 2003], a practice that can also be found in educational institutions that developed an anti-discrimination protocol [Vedder, Bouwer & Pels, 1996].

In stress-coping models, discrimination is seen as a stressor. If stress is accumulating and coping opportunities are limited, the stress may start to negatively impact on a person's physical and mental health [cf. Brondolo, ver Halen, Pencille, Beatty & Contrada, 2009]. Particularly stressors that are uncontrollable and unpredictable, like discrimination, considerably add to the risk of mental and physical health damages

[Williams & Mohammed, 2009]. Most research that we presented or summarized in the introductory section used measures of perceived discrimination and was not specific to educational settings. Pascoe and Richman [2009] conducted a meta-analytic review of research on perceived discrimination and health. Although they not only and specifically focused on school-related perceived discrimination, their findings also are valid for school-related perceived discrimination. They concluded that through stress reactions and its impact on health behaviors, perceived discrimination is likely to have a negative impact on children's and adolescents' well-being and health.

## Coping with Discrimination

Brondolo et al. [2009] reviewed research on three forms of coping with racism: development of a strong racial identity, social support seeking, and anger suppression and expression.

*Ethnic Identity and Self-Esteem*
In the introduction, we already referred to a strong and positive ethnic identity development as a coping strategy when speaking about the rejection identification model [Branscombe et al., 1999] which suggests that as a reaction to discrimination, people will choose to identify themselves more strongly as a member of their own group. How a strong ethnic identity protects a person against the negative consequences of discrimination experiences is not very clear [Brondolo et al., 2009], but it seems important to consider ethnic identity both as an individual characteristic and as a social one [Phinney, Horenczyk, Liebkind & Vedder, 2001]. Ethnic identity as an individual characteristic may allow persons who are confident in their own ethnicity and proud of their ethnic group to deal more constructively with discrimination. They may do so by regarding discrimination as the problem of the perpetrator or the system, or by taking proactive steps to combat discrimination [Berry et al., 2006b]. Noh, Beiser, Kaspar, Hou and Rummens [1999] even suggest that a strong ethnic orientation may stimulate or facilitate the use of forbearance as a means to limit the negative impact of discrimination experiences.

Phinney, Horenczyk, Liebkind & Vedder [2001] define ethnic identity as that aspect of acculturation which focuses on the subjective sense of belonging to a group or culture. Stated differently, they consider ethnic identity in the context of acculturation, or the context of changes that take shape at the individual and social level due to continued contact between different groups. They do so, because it is the process of acculturation in which ethnic identity becomes salient and more important. The salience is manifested in combating feelings of despair about discrimination and harassment experienced personally or as a group, but also in feelings of connectedness, solidarity and security when solidarity and connectedness are seen as or experienced as effective instruments against discrimination and harassment, meaning that ethnic identity and its adaptive function depend on context and experiences. Where there is pressure to assimilate, and immigrants are willing to adapt to the new culture, and resources are available, national identity should be predictive of positive outcomes. When there is a strong supportive ethnic community, along with a positive contextual reception, a strong ethnic identity should predict positive outcomes. In such a situation, ethnic identity represents a proxy for a social support system that buffers against or alleviates the consequences of discrimination experiences. Moreover, a vital ethnic community provides a context in which children can form a positive sense of their group and of themselves [Liebkind & Jasinskaja-Lahti, 2000]. This is reflected in a secure sense of one's ethnicity, which is a source of personal strength and positive self-evaluation [Phinney & Kohatsu, 1997]. The combination of the two (a robust sense of the group and sense of oneself as a member of that community) creates

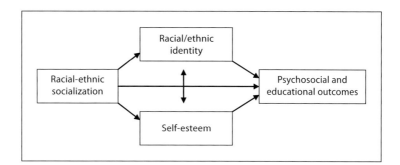

**Fig. 1.** Ethnic identity and self-esteem as explanation for the relationship between ethnic socialization and adaptation outcomes.

conditions that allow an individual to see an act of discrimination not so much as an act against the person, but as an act against the group. The burden of discrimination is carried by many, which makes it easier to forbear it [Mossakowski, 2003]. Apart from the support of the community and this notion of sharing the burden of discrimination, a strong ethnic sense of self and a strong ethnic self-esteem may weaken or neutralize the impact of discrimination experiences, like protective factors counterbalance or frustrate the working of risk factors in psychopathology.

The social aspect of ethnic identity is also stressed in developmental notions of ethnic identity. Children who are exposed to negative stereotypes about their own group may hold conflicting or negative feelings about their ethnicity [Phinney, 1989]. However, children are also influenced by messages received from the family and community [Knight et al., 1993; Vedder, Berry, Sabatier & Sam, 2009]. Parental socialization regarding ethnicity plays an important role in the content and meaning children attach to their own ethnicity [Bernal et al., 1990; Hughes, Witherspoon, Rivas-Drake & West-Bey, 2009; Thornton, Chatters, Taylor & Allen, 1990]. How this works in relation to socialization efforts aimed at sheltering children for the negative consequences of discrimination was explored by Rodriguez, Umaña-Taylor, Smith and Johnson [2009]. They tested the following model (fig. 1).

This model [adapted after Hughes et al., 2009] expresses the notion that the relationship between racial or ethnic socialization and psychosocial and educational outcomes is mediated by self-system processes like self-esteem and ethnic identity. Rodriguez et al. [2009] reviewed research testing this model. They concluded that it is useful to distinguish socialization practices using cultural pride messages from practices that prepare children for discrimination. The first practice coincides with higher levels of self-esteem and ethnic identity and also in stronger beliefs in one's own academic competencies. The second approach was associated with lower levels of self-esteem, more doubts about one's ethnic identity and minor behavioral problems [cf. Hughes et al., 2009], which suggests that the explicit attention for discrimination raised the fear and alertness for such experiences [Cohen & Garcia, 2005]. Interestingly, a combined use of both practices had the same positive outcomes as cultural pride messages. Brondolo et al. [2009] qualify the positive interpretations of the role of cultural pride. Cultural pride makes a person's ethnic identity more important to the person, and this so-called raised sense of the centrality of ethnic identity may eventually, like explicit attention for discrimination, fuel fear of discrimination. This seems to primarily result in distress and depression.

In sum, ethnic identity either as a referent to a strong self-esteem or as a marker to the availability of social support (from family or the ethnic group) may help in protecting persons from the negative consequences of discrimination experiences. However, if the attention for ethnic identity is accompanied by an increasing fear of discrimination, the consequences turn from positive to negative. Whether this actually will happen depends on a multitude of possible person-context interactions of which we gave some examples. However, as pointed out by Brondolo et al. [2009], most available studies used correlational designs and hence do not allow for cause-effect reasoning.

*Social Support*

The second possible coping strategy for dealing with discrimination is social support seeking. While discussing the possible role of ethnic identity as a buffer against discrimination experiences, we already contended that a strong ethnic identity may be indicative of the availability of social support, which may involve direct communication, sharing experiences or the perception and anticipation of support, knowing that one is covered and can count on others. The review by Brondolo et al. [2009] clarifies that there is scant support from quantitative studies for the positive role of social support when persons are confronted with discrimination although, again, the available studies are mostly correlational in nature. These studies suggest that when persons' exposure to stressors is low, and social support is perceived as available, this perception coincides with less health risks (for instance, lower blood pressure). This suggests that social support might have a buffering function against discrimination for health risks. However, from the available studies it is not possible to conclude whether or not the relationships discussed are causal or not. Such a conclusion needs further research. In addition to this design-related qualification, Brondolo et al. [2009] also clarify that studies on sharing grave discrimination experiences show that victims may react with very strong emotional distress and anger due to recollections or experiences of reviving episodes of harassment. In addition, sharing discrimination experiences may raise the fear of it happening again. So, if indeed new research shows a causal link between sharing discrimination experiences and negative adaptation or health outcomes, we already have a notion of its explanation, viz. recollection of or reviving episodes of harassment and fear of repetition.

What we know about social support and its buffering effects for discrimination experiences is simply too little. We have no idea about the validity of particular models across gender, SES, cultural or age groups or how they are related to particular developmental stages and, in the case of children, the quality of educational settings and relationships. With respect to children, studies conducted by Jasinskaja-Lahti and Liebkind [2001] and Liebkind, Jasinskaja-Lahti and Solheim [2004] seem to lead to more positive conclusions. They studied the role of parental support as a buffer against discrimination for immigrant adolescents. A higher level of parental support was related to lower levels of perceived discrimination. The explanation suggested by the authors was that when confronted with host majority discrimination, immigrant adults can help children to rationalize, or clarify the reasons behind the discrimination, which helps the children to attribute the discrimination to characteristics of the discriminating persons, not to characteristics of the discriminated. Whether indeed adolescents talk to their parents about these issues was not explored in those two studies. It may be that just being supported at home protects children from stress. This way, a positive self-image can be maintained. Young immigrants in particular may not be able to understand and deal with the associated negative feelings constructively and the reasons behind experiences with discrimination and thus be reliant on social and psychological support provided by their parents. Actually, a focus on parental support may be too limited. Effects of availability and use of ethnic peer networks, national peer networks and networks abroad have also been suggested to have a buffering effect on the relation between perceived discrimination and cognitive and emotional outcomes [Jasinskaja-Lahti, Liebkind, Jaakkola & Reuter, 2006].

With respect to children, particularly students, it seems wise to also have a look at a comparable domain, viz. bullying. A variety of scholars [Mooney, Creeser & Blatchford, 1991; Olweus, 1997] suggest a similarity between bullying and racism, which is the belief that race determines human traits and capacities and that a particular race is superior, and justifies the oppression or abuse of representatives of other races. Both bullying and racism are examples of intentional harm, unprovoked by the victims, linked to a perceived imbalance of power between perpetrators and victims. A possible difference is that racism is a depreciation of all aspects of other persons, and thus has no age limits, whereas bullying may be instigated by particular characteristics or activities (e.g. weight, wearing glasses) [cf. Mooney et al., 1991], and is normally limited to peers. Often, friends are similar in ethnic background [Graham & Cohen, 1997; McPherson, Smith-Lovin & Cook, 2001]. Perhaps more importantly, immigrant youth with friends from similar ethnic backgrounds are less open to members of other ethnic groups than youth who have inter-ethnic friends [Phinney, Romero, Nava & Huang, 2001]. Such results suggest that ethnicity serves as a valued characteristic for friendship selection, and at the same time as a powerful selective socializing agent and potential source or bases for discrimination. An important research finding [Bellmore, Witkow, Graham & Juvonen, 2004] stresses the importance of whether a student belongs to a minority or a majority group. Being rejected (or being discriminated against) while belonging to the majority has stronger negative effects on a student's well-being than being rejected while belonging to the minority. The criterion for minority or majority may vary. It can refer to racial classification, ethnicity, religion, economic prosperity and many other characteristics, some of which may be politically charged. In any case, the most likely explanation for this finding is that children who belong to the majority group in a class or school are, given the earlier presented research on in-group bias, likely to perceive or anticipate support from within this group, and hence are more disappointed about being harassed and not receiving any support. In short, it is not just a matter of receiving support or not, but also from whom or more importantly from whom not.

*Anger Suppression and Expression*
The third way of coping with discrimination to be dealt with here is anger suppression and expression or acceptance and confrontation. Suppression is meant to let the negative feeling or the distress caused by experiencing discrimination pass by, 'get it over with' in the hope that it stops or at least not intensifies. Anger expression or confrontation is meant to get in control, either to influence the gravity or extent of the damage and stop the harassment or to stay on top of the strong emotions triggered by the perpetrator and the shame and doubt the discrimination causes (loss of face). Brondolo et al. [2009] show that relatively few studies have been conducted to analyze the value of these coping strategies. They report that the available studies show that expressing anger as compared to suppressing it seems to covary with lower risks of health problems and depression. Suppressing anger does not help people when they experience discrimination. The explanation for the findings is actually different from what we suggested in the opening lines of this paragraph; suppression does not lead to 'getting it over with', but instead leads to rumination of the experiences, and hence to prolongation of the stress. Confrontation on the other hand may stop the harassment, and may also boost one's self-esteem. As Brondolo et al. [2009] rightfully pointed out, there is still a long way to go between the available research findings and a recommendation or even a training program aimed at supporting young persons to confront acts of discrimination. We have no

systematic knowledge of possible moderators like age, gender and ethnicity of offended and perpetrator or of the interaction between these characteristics of offended and perpetrator. Neither do we know what contexts or time of day would allow for the use of a confrontation strategy without running the risk of reprisals. Could it be that the risk of physical assault is bigger when there are few other persons around or a crowd that backs the perpetrator, and that downtown Washington DC is a safer place for confrontation during daylight and on working days than at night and during the weekend? We may assume the answers, but actually they are not research based.

This abridged version of a summary of research findings on coping with discrimination or racism leaves us with the notion that we need more research for a clearer picture of effective coping strategies. The bleak picture that is now visible suggests that pride of one's ethnic culture, a strong self-esteem based on trust in the own family members and community as a secure environment, together with a functional approach aimed at stopping or regulating discrimination and its negative impact are the beacons that should allow us to steer clear of racism, discrimination and their negative consequences.

**Multicultural Education and Discrimination**

In the preceding sections, we have clarified that in culturally diverse communities, people may be confronted with discrimination, prejudice and culture-related harassment. Moreover, although we have not exclusively focused on children in our review, it is clear that children also are affected by discrimination. This is particularly clear from studies on schools and discrimination. By discussing studies on coping strategies, we have put steps towards resolving the problems that emerge as a consequence of experiencing discrimination. In the remainder of this chapter we will focus more on children, or more particularly on students (children and adolescents). We will consider schools as the ideal place to do something about prejudice, discrimination and their consequences. In doing so, we will pay attention to prejudice and discrimination in school, but also to discrimination before children go to school and during out of school hours. Those are all experiences that may impact the way students feel and behave while in school. Moreover, schools are supposed to prepare children for their further social participation for now as well as for the future. Schools have a responsibility in dealing with discrimination and teaching children how to cope with discrimination and more generally stated, with the uncertainty and tensions that have evolved in interethnic relationships, because not all children and their parents can cope equally well with cultural diversity. In short, it makes sense to approach the topic of discrimination and schools from three perspectives: (a) discrimination as a social problem, (b) schooling as a process of discrimination, in which the school, by using particular didactical approaches and assessment and differentiation strategies, affirms and contributes to social inequality in society, and (c) schools as a place where students and teachers meet and some individuals and groups experience discrimination.

Using the first perspective, schools are given the responsibility or task to deal with a broad social problem that has consequences for how students and teachers interact and how students and teachers perform their tasks and how they feel about it. The second perspective focuses on variations in well-being and academic achievements between cultural groups in school that can be explained by bias in curricular materials, tests, assessment and teaching strategies, and teachers' attitudes and styles of communication with students [Vedder & Horenczyk, 2006]. The third perspective is the one most clearly represented in the preceding section. It focuses on teachers' and students' experiences of discrimination and how they cope with those experiences. It is primarily about subjective interpretations and the accompanying feelings.

The first two perspectives are also characterized by more or less clear notions of the causes of discrimination. For instance, Social Identity Theory fits the first perspective. Social Identity Theory [Tajfel & Turner, 1986] teaches us that it is beneficial for boosting one's self esteem to be a member of a group that with respect to particular characteristics or achievements is valued more than other groups. To achieve this boost in self-esteem persons have to distinguish groups, try to belong to the group in highest esteem and when needed or beneficial, support the definition as well as the maintenance of group boundaries, even if it takes the use of prejudice and discrimination. The theory describes that enhancing one's self-esteem is an important motive for discrimination. For the sake of qualification, it is worthwhile commenting that the theory does not state that anyone can choose membership in all groups she or he would want to. Sometimes persons do not have a choice and feel frustrated or are forced to join a group and cannot pass and feel frustrated.

Another source of discrimination is even more basic, viz. intergenerational and intragenerational transmission. Allport [1954], Milner [1983], Holmes [1995], and more recently Liebkind [2006] reminds us that children are born into families that try hard to make sure that children learn and represent the same values as parents and other family members. They model preferred behaviors including discrimination between the own and other groups, including ethnic groups. Holmes [1995] even hints at the community as a source of modeled discrimination in that discrimination is aimed at those persons who do not behave or who do not have the looks in accordance with a common majority standard. Vedder, Berry, Sabatier and Sam [2009] showed that questions like 'Are our children behaving the way their peers do?' or 'Are our children behaving the way other adults want them to?' guide parents in their behavior towards their children. If the answer is no, then parents may decide to interfere and regulate with whom their children interact, hence they model discrimination.

In the description of the second perspective, the causes of discrimination were already identified: the school and all instruments used in schools may jeopardize the developmental opportunities of particular groups of students to do well in school. It is beyond the scope of this chapter to specify how from each of these perspectives, schools can deal with all discrimination-related phenomena that have been described so far. In what follows we will be selective. We focus on a goal that is common to all three perspectives. From all three perspectives, policy makers, parents, teachers, and students can draw inspiration to state that schools are responsible for improving the quality of interethnic or intercultural relationships in order to stop discrimination and prejudice. Apart from this attention for the improvement of the quality of interethnic relationships, we will focus on the third perspective and two coping strategies that were presented earlier.

*Improving Interethnic Relationships*

Intergroup contact is considered to be an effective strategy for improving intergroup relationships and for solving problems related to ethnocultural diversity. As school and other educational institutions are traditionally viewed as major arenas for intergroup contact and acculturation, they are perceived to be of great importance for improving interethnic relationships [Vedder, Horenzyk & Liebkind, 2006]. With regard to ethnicity, research shows that children mostly choose friends with the same ethnic background [see above, Graham & Cohen, 1997; Tatum, 2003], and from this it is easily concluded that there are only very limited inter-ethnic interactions in classes. However, studies that do compare friendships with interaction networks find contradicting results as to the role of ethnicity within these relations. Denscombe, Szulc, Patrick and Wood [1986] found few interethnic friendships in elementary classrooms but plenty of interethnic social interaction during breaks. In an older group of Caribbean English adolescents, Reynolds [2007] found that while best friends were also Caribbean, the larger social networks consisted of people from a wide range of ethnic backgrounds. However, Aboud, Mendelson and Purdy [2003] reported that while elementary school children had more same- than cross-race companions (interaction partners), only older children (grade 5 or 6) had more same- than cross-race friends. When looking at second and fifth grade students, Aboud and Sankar [2007] also found that students had more intraethnic than interethnic interaction companions, but surprisingly equivalent numbers of friends from both groups. The latter seems more generally the case when looking at studies on interethnic friendship relationships that corrected for the opportunity to interact with students from various backgrounds. The proportion of interethnic friendships of minority group students became similar to the proportion of interethnic friendships of national students [Aboud et al., 2003; Baerveldt, Van Duijn, Vermeij & Van Hemert, 2004]. With or without this correction, however, the conclusion is that both immigrant students [Kao & Vaquera, 2006; Titzmann, Silbereisen & Schmitt-Rodermund, 2007] and national students [Kao & Joyner, 2004] show a preference for intraethnic friendships and have predominantly ethnically homogeneous peer networks.

Several models and theories present mechanisms of influencing or regulating intergroup relationships. The Common In-group Identity Model [Gaertner & Dovidio, 2000] seeks to influence the perception of group boundaries by manipulating persons' experience or perception of intergroup contact situations. The manipulation is inspired by a related model, the social categorization theory that represents the notion that people are categorized into groups that can vary in terms of inclusiveness, and that categories can be reconsidered and persons recategorized [Gaunt, 2009]. Recategorization may be geared at combining initially separate groups into one group by using a common superordinate category. Since after the recategorization the outgroup no longer exists as such, earlier negative feelings and interactions diminish. Recategorization can be triggered by showing how it is done and by showing that it can be a rewarding experience. Quintana, Castaneda-English and Ybarra [1999] suggested that in the context of intercultural relationships recategorization has primarily to do with regulating cognitive processes, learning how to reason logically and not with ethnic socialization. Thus in order for children to be able to recategorize group memberships of themselves or other persons, they primarily would need cognitive training or, more generally, the development of cognitive competences. Socialization geared at celebrating cultural diversity or at acquiring better knowledge of ethnic differences and their significance in particular communities would not support the desired recategorization competence. Pettigrew [1998] described the process of recategorization as one in which initial categorization leads in contact situations to fear reactions and a confirmation of the categorization ('I am a Christian and you are a Muslim; I don't like you.'). If the contact lasts and leads to positive feelings about the contact this leads to de-categorization ('Well . . ., you are a Muslim, but nevertheless a nice person'; a process of de-categorization takes shape, without being replaced by a new generalization). The label 'nice person' is exclusively meant for one person. Prolonged contact that is enjoyed by all persons involved, combined with an awareness that these persons represent larger groups such as Christians and Muslims leads to less prejudice and discrimination in which the initial categorization (Christian, Muslim) plays a role and eventually leads to a recategorization ('You are a Christian, but what is more important to me is that we, you and I, have a lot in common and are good friends. Most likely I could be good friends with many other Christians as well.')

A more popular model in de educational arena is the intergroup contact theory [Allport, 1954]. It suggests that prolonged contact between ethnic groups may reduce prejudice if the contact satisfies particular conditions. Groups must enter the contact situation with equal status, there must be cooperative interdependence between the groups, and the contact must occur in the context of supportive norms. Dovidio, Gaertner and Kawakami [2003] suggest that in order for social contact to be effective, the category membership of the individuals in the interaction must be of at least minimal salience. Hence, they link the contact theory and the social categorization theory. This minimal salience is necessary in order to ensure the generalization from the positive contact with one or a couple of outgroup members to the improved intergroup attitudes to the outgroup as a whole [Dovidio et al., 2003]. Pettigrew and Tropp [2006] commented that acquaintance and friendship take time to occur and have an impact. They therefore define time of exposure between members of different groups as an additional important feature of efforts to improve intergroup relations. Indeed, studies show that organizing learning in well-structured cooperative learning groups in which students vary in cultural backgrounds but share common goals and are interdependent in achieving these goals, makes for improved relationships between students across ethnic boundaries [Oortwijn, Boekaerts, Vedder & Fortuin, 2008].

Another likely way to improve the quality and intensity of interethnic relationships is by improving the school climate. School climate deals with relationships amongst classmates and between students and teachers. School climate may refer to experiences and interactions that take shape in classrooms, but also in hallways, the playground or in cafeterias. It is about feeling safe, respected and challenged to be active and learn respected and appreciated things and achieving both teacher set and personal learning and developmental goals. To further clarify this, we once more take a look at research on bullying. The school climate covaries with the occurrence of bullying, harassment or discrimination. Olweus [1993] and with him Rigby [2008] suggest that a better school climate makes students feel respected and confident and that their school is a good, safe place to be. In such a climate, the students will feel less frustrated and bored and will engage less in bullying or harassing peers [Rigby, 2008].

Not all teachers may be equally interested or certain about dealing with harassment and discrimination, its reduction or prevention. Teacher's uncertainty or unwillingness to deal with discrimination invites students who discriminate or harass to continue their aggression towards their peers and it confuses the victims and bystanders, who, as a consequence, will not report the incidents to the teacher. This is the more serious as we realize that maximizing the responsibility or role of the teacher for reducing discrimination and its negative consequences is likely to be the most effective intervention in school if they act decisively and consistently, and carefully plan their activities, e.g. for supervising activities and places where students meet, possibly in collaboration with other teachers [Kochenderfer-Ladd & Pelletier, 2008]. Moreover, schools would be well advised to monitor school climate regularly and discuss the outcomes with students, parents/guardians and teachers to explore the need and opportunities to improve the school climate.

*Ethnic Identity and Support*
The notion of school climate is closely linked to two of the coping strategies discussed earlier: ethnic identity and support. Vollmer [2000] has indicated that teachers' beliefs have a strong influence on a schools' educational and social climate. When a teacher is dealing with a culturally diverse group of students, his/her preferences about how students should feel about and behave with respect to their own ethnic and to the national culture may influence the students in several ways. A teacher that prefers the immigrant

students to take over the values and customs typical of the new society of settlement and deny or neglect their own ethnic culture may discourage immigrant students to explore their cultural identities, inclusive of speaking their native language in school. Moreover, the teacher may communicate, more or less explicitly, to the national students that they are in the good team. By doing so, the teacher is narrowing the immigrant students' possibilities for integration, by denying them their wish for establishing and maintaining links with both the ethnic and the national culture. From the perspective of the national students, the teacher signals that there is no need for them to be interested in the immigrant students' cultural background. After all, it is neither useful nor valued, and it is just transitional.

This is not good for immigrant children's ethnic identity exploration and development and certainly not conducive to positive, threat-free interactions or positive relationships across ethnic groups. Many studies suggest that an integrationist attitude, which is combining the ethnic cultural maintenance with participation in the national culture, in students coincides with the best chances of a healthy development [Berry et al., 2006a]. Moreover, the interactive model of acculturation [Bourhis, Moise, Perreault & Senecal, 1997] clarifies that different expectations regarding acculturation attitudes between immigrants and nationals may create tension and even conflict. Thus, even though integration is often found conducive to immigrant health, it may produce tense relations between immigrants and nationals if nationals are not supportive of immigrants' cultural maintenance.

There are two more important consequences. Research by Tatar and Horenczyk [2003] shows that teachers who work with culturally diverse classes and are not appreciative of immigrant students' cultural background and, instead, want them to assimilate the national, normative values and customs as swiftly as possible, run a high risk of stress and stress-related health problems. In short, they cannot function optimally as teachers. This will also impair their willingness and capacity to support students who experience discrimination. These same researchers [Horenczyk & Tatar, 1998] also showed that normally immigrant children know that they have to learn how to behave in their new cultural environment. In their effort to get to know the new society and how to move in it, they tend to think very positively about peers of the national group as resources, guides and supporters in their effort. Teachers' attitudes towards cultural diversity and immigrant children's cultural backgrounds can make it more difficult for immigrant children to establish the desired contacts with national peers. After all, and as clarified before, being presented consciously or unconsciously by teachers as culturally non-normative or deficient is likely to fuel prejudice and discrimination in national students. If this happens, calling on these same peers to assist in coping with discrimination experiences is also likely to be extremely difficult, if not impossible.

A school with a strong multicultural policy may help to reduce the problems outlined above. We define multicultural education based on Parekhs' [2002] work as education entailing respect for cultural differences as resources for learning and development amongst both teachers and students. Implementing a model of dual language learning provides an example of a school not only celebrating the reading of stories but also the oral tradition of story telling [cf. May, 1994; Zentella, 2005]. Tatar and Horenczyk [2003] report those teachers who support this notion and transmit it to their students experience less stress as a result of interaction with immigrant students than colleagues who consider it school's as well as their own exclusive task to introduce students to mainstream society. Furthermore, in an experimental study by Richeson and Nussbaum [2004] it was found that individuals that endorse multicultural attitudes have a lower racial bias than individuals that endorse color-blindness.

# A Study on the Effects of School Multiculturalism

In the preceding sections, we reviewed the effects of discrimination on health. We furthermore argued that school is a place where discrimination may take place, but that creating a multicultural atmosphere in the school might help to reduce discrimination. In this section, we will demonstrate empirically that a more multicultural atmosphere in schools is related to less discrimination and a higher well-being among immigrant adolescents. In the previous sections, we provided an intricate and complex description of discrimination and ways to deal with it. In the empirical study that follows, we shall use simpler operationalizations of discrimination and multicultural education. Earlier, we referred to three perspectives on the relationship between school and discrimination. We will use here the third perspective: schools dealing with perceived discrimination. In this chapter, we have outlined that for avoiding and combating discrimination schools can focus on a broad variety of measures, and as such it will be difficult to capture all in a single empirical study. We will show that neither discrimination nor multicultural education need to be considered in their full complexity in order for a study to clarify the potential of schools to do something about discrimination. Even with crude indications of discrimination, its effects on mental and physical health become apparent [Paradies, 2006]. Similarly, even small subaspects of multicultural education such as teachers talking about discrimination have been found effective in reducing discrimination in the classroom [Verkuyten & Thijs, 2002]. The goal of this study is to demonstrate how students' evaluation of their schools' multicultural climate may already be related to experienced discrimination and well-being among immigrant students. With that purpose in mind, we chose to study a sample of Muslim immigrant adolescents in the Netherlands. Many Dutch nationals are prejudiced towards Muslims [Gonzalez, Verkuyten, Weesie & Poppe, 2008], and Muslims are more likely than any other religious group in the Netherlands to become the victims of hate crimes [Wagenaar & Van Donselaar, 2008].

## Method

*Sample*

Our sample consisted of 155 Muslim immigrant adolescents. Ages ranged from 12 to 16, the mean age was 13.74 years (SD = 1.08). The sample consisted of 91 boys and 64 girls. Of the respondents, 41 were born outside the Netherlands (first generation) and 114 had at least one parent born outside the Netherlands (second generation). The sample was gathered at four junior vocational high schools in the western part of the Netherlands, the main city area between Amsterdam and Rotterdam, and spread out over 26 classrooms. Muslim immigrants in the Netherlands are mostly of Turkish or Moroccan origin. Many Turkish and Moroccan immigrants came to the Netherlands during the 1960s as guest laborers, and built up a life for themselves there. Muslim immigrants often live in ethnic enclaves [Phalet & Schönpflug, 2001]. Studies on the acculturation attitudes of both Turkish [Arends-Toth & Van de Vijver, 2003], and Moroccan [Ouarasse & van de Vijver, 2005] immigrants reveal that most prefer integration (i.e. combining the wish to maintain ones cultural identity and seeking active ways to participate in the majority, national or host community) into the Dutch society.

*Instruments*

Self-reports were used for the purpose of this study. Questionnaires started with questions concerning the respondents' place of birth, parents' place of birth, religion, age and gender. The perceived discrimination, behavioral problems, psychological problems and self-esteem scales were taken from the ICSEY study [Berry et al., 2006a]. Our motivation scale was based on the scale developed by Ryan and Deci [2000]. For the purpose of this study, we developed a scale to measure students' perceptions of multicultural atmosphere in the school. The scale consisted of three items, namely 'In my school it is assumed that cultural maintenance will help me to succeed', 'In my school ethnic and cultural diversity is respected', and 'In my school we are taught to respect ethnic and cultural differences'. All items were rated on a five-point scale ranging from completely agree to completely disagree. Means, standard deviations and Cronbach's alphas of the scales are reported in table 1.

**Table 1.** Means, standard deviations and Cronbach's alphas for the variables in this study

|  | Mean | SD | Cronbach's alpha |
|---|---|---|---|
| Discrimination | 2.35 | 0.76 | 0.69 |
| School multiculturalism | 3.55 | 0.87 | 0.74 |
| Motivation | 3.27 | 0.70 | 0.69 |
| Behavioral problems | 1.84 | 0.78 | 0.84 |
| Self-esteem | 3.86 | 0.60 | 0.73 |
| Psychological problems | 2.07 | 0.75 | 0.84 |

## Results

*School Differences in Discrimination and Multicultural Atmosphere*

To analyze whether students' experiences with discrimination and evaluations of school multiculturalism were attributable to the school, we computed intraclass correlation coefficients (school level variance divided by total variance). It was found that 18% of the variation in students' experiences with discrimination and 35% of students' evaluation of the schools' multicultural atmosphere can be explained at the school level. Although only four schools are included in this analysis, this suggests that the experience of discrimination can not be explained solely at the individual level: Muslim students' reports of discrimination are in part related to the school they attend.

*Relations between Perceived School Multicultural Atmosphere, Discrimination and Well-Being*

The model depicted in figure 2 was fitted to the data using a path analysis. In this model, the relations between students' perceptions of the schools' multicultural atmosphere and adaptation outcomes are mediated by perceived discrimination, but we also modeled direct relations between the perceptions of multicultural atmosphere and adaptation outcomes (as such it is a partially mediated model). We used a maximum likelihood estimation procedure to evaluate model fit. Based on previous literature [i.e. Steinberg et al., 1992], we modeled relations between the adaptation outcomes. Because the relations between these variables have already been well established, and because their inter-relations are not the purpose of this study, we have not included their regression weights in figure 2 (table 2). Overall, the model showed excellent fit [$\chi^2$ (1, n = 145) = 1.879, p < 0.05; SRMR = 0.02; CFI = 1.00; GFI = 1.00]. The standardized regression weights are included in figure 2. Although not all the relations between perceived discrimination, perceptions of multicultural atmosphere and adaptation were significant, in general the model fit and regression weights support the notion that creating a multicultural atmosphere in the school may help to reduce discrimination and increase well-being among immigrant students.

## Discussion

The goal of the study was to analyze whether a schools' perceived multicultural atmosphere would coincide with fewer reports of discrimination and a higher well-being amongst Islamic immigrant adolescents. Consistent with previous research [e.g. Berry et al., 2006a; Jasinskaja-Lahti & Liebkind, 2001; Verkuyten, 1998] it was found

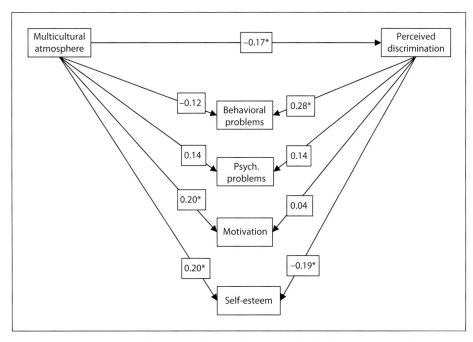

**Fig. 2.** The model that was fitted to the data, including standardized regression weights.

**Table 2.** Correlations between multicultural atmosphere, discrimination and the outcome variables motivation, behavioral problems, self-esteem and behavioral problems

|  | Multiculturalism | Discrimination | Motivation | Behavioral problems | Self-esteem |
|---|---|---|---|---|---|
| Discrimination | −0.18* | | | | |
| Motivation | 0.22** | −0.02 | | | |
| Behavioral problems | −0.23** | 0.35** | −0.33** | | |
| Self-esteem | 0.23** | −0.21** | 0.12 | −0.19* | |
| Psychological problems | 0.01 | 0.22** | −0.14 | 0.30** | −0.39** |

* p < 0.05; ** p < 0.01.

that perceived discrimination had negative relations with adolescents' self-esteem and was related to more behavioral problems; however, we found no relations with psychological problems and motivation. It may be that the relations between psychological problems and discrimination reported in previous studies [e.g., Berry et al., 2006] may be mediated by self-esteem.

Earlier, we presented the school both as a risk and as a place of opportunity in this regard. In our analyses, it was found that 18% of the variance in student-reported discrimination was attributable to the school level. This suggests that in some schools students are more likely to report feelings of discrimination than in other schools, and stresses the importance of developing interventions at the school level.

At the school level, 35% of students' evaluation of the schools' multicultural atmosphere could be explained. We do not know how students come to evaluate the schools' multicultural atmosphere as they do, but the sizeable explained variance at the school level suggests that students experience differences in schools' multicultural atmospheres. Some schools in the Netherlands may be more willing or more successful at implementing multicultural policies. It would be useful if in future studies, the school multicultural atmosphere could be measured through direct observations or independent reports.

The importance of having multicultural schools is demonstrated by these results. Not only was the schools' multicultural atmosphere related to lower reports of discrimination, it was also related to a better motivation and higher self-esteem amongst Islamic immigrant students. Research already indicates that cultural maintenance among immigrant students may help them to thrive academically [Fuligni, 1998] and experience a more positive well-being [Van Geel & Vedder, 2011], and as such it is not surprising that a school that allows for cultural maintenance is related to a higher well-being among immigrant students. Multiculturalism is about acknowledging and respecting. Although the meaning of the term multiculturalism may be debated, basically it means that cultural diversity is not only respected but also valued [Parekh, 2002]. This combination of respecting and valuing cultural diversity may explain why school multiculturalism is related to fewer reports of discrimination.

*Limitations*
Unfortunately, we were only able to acquire self-reports, and research suggests that discrepancies may exist between student reports of well-being, and teacher and parent reports [Stevens, Pels, Bengi-Arslan, Verhulst, Vollebergh & Crijnen, 2003]. We do not have longitudinal data, and as such we can only speculate about cause and effect relations. Finally, the data presented in this study would typically be tested using a multilevel model. However, the schools, classrooms and the respondents are too few to meaningfully analyze with a multilevel model. We focused our study on Muslim immigrants in the Netherlands, and the findings will need to be reproduced in other samples to establish in how far the results are generalizable across immigrant and age groups.

*Implications*
Despite the limitations, this study holds several important implications. Few empirical studies exist regarding the effects of school multiculturalism on immigrant students. This study suggests that multiculturalism in schools is related to both discrimination and student well-being, and as such future studies are warranted. The more important implications are at the school level however. It has been found that teachers view the assimilation of immigrant students as one of their important educational tasks. Ironically, the most assimilative teachers were found to suffer stronger degrees of burnout [Tatar & Horenczyk, 2003]. Our study suggests that this motivation of teachers to assimilate students may be severely at odds with immigrant students' needs, as they seem to do best in a multicultural school.

The sheer fact that ethnically diverse schools are characterized by a student body made up of students with diverse cultural background is akin to the contention that such schools are ideal places for discrimination. Although Parekh [2002] states that cultural diversity may be enriching to ones' life, the state of ethnic diversity in high schools indicates that some management may be required if ethnic diversity is really going to be an asset. The teachers and other adults may play a key role in creating a multicultural school. However, they would need to be made aware of the negative effects of discrimination, and the benefits of multiculturalism. Next to awareness, teachers would also need the necessary tools to create multicultural schools. A study by Verkuyten and Thijs [2002] indicates that a teacher that talks about discrimination and ethnic diversity may already reduce discrimination in their classrooms. Increased contact and cooperation [Allport, 1954; Pettigrew, 1998; Sherif, 1966] may also do much to improve interethnic relations in the school. However, future studies should indicate how multicultural schools may be created most effectively. With increasing numbers of immigrants into western society [Suarez-Orozco, 2001], such knowledge will become increasingly important.

## Conclusions

Ideally, schools in culturally diverse societies would prepare students for participation in that diverse society. If they are not inspired by this challenge, the least they can do is to provide a safe learning environment in which all students, regardless of culture or ethnicity, can thrive. In a world that is increasingly ethnically diverse, this means that interethnic relations need to be managed, and that the well-being of immigrant students needs to be considered. Many teachers hold assimilationist views, or show no interest in cultural diversity. However, strong efforts on the teachers' part to assimilate immigrant students may send the message to national students that immigrant students have an inferior culture, and as such teachers may contribute to interethnic tensions. Furthermore, by forcing immigrant students to assimilate, immigrant students may be robbed of cultural traits that may help them succeed in education, and they may be denied the chance to develop a positive ethnic identity, a valuable buffer against experiences of discrimination. As outlined in this chapter, discrimination at schools happens at different levels, and some forms of discrimination are deeply rooted in society, and as such we do not mean to convey the message that there is an easy cure. However, as our review and analyses indicate, a school and classrooms in which cultural diversity is respected may already reduce interpersonal discrimination and promote more positive interethnic relations. In order to achieve schools with positive multicultural atmospheres, teachers need to play an active and key role. Teachers are a decisive influence on the school climate, and it is likely that the teachers' attitude towards ethnic diversity will have a strong influence on the interethnic relations in school.

## References

Aboud, F.E., Mendelson, M.J., & Purdy, K.T. (2003). Cross-race peer relations and friendship quality. *International Journal of Behavioral Development, 27,* 165–173.

Aboud, F.E., & Sankar, J. (2007). Friendship and identity in a language-integrated school. *International Journal of Behavioral Development, 31,* 445–453.

Akerlof, G., & Kranton, R. (2002). Identity and schooling: Some lessons for the economics of education, *Journal of Economic Literature, 40,* 1167–1201.

Allport, G. (1954). *The nature of prejudice.* Garden City: Doubleday Anchor Books.

Arends-Toth, T., & Van de Vijver, F.J.R. (2003). Multiculturalism and acculturation: Views of Dutch and Turkish-Dutch. *European Journal of Social Psychology, 33,* 249–266.

Baerveldt, C., van Duijn, M.A.J., Vermeij, L., & van Hemert, D.A. (2004). Ethnic boundaries and personal choice. Assessing the influence of individual inclinations to choose intra-ethnic relationships on pupils' networks. *Social Networks. An International Journal of Structural Analysis, 26,* 55–74.

Bellmore, A.D., Witkow, M.R., Graham, S., & Juvonen, J. (2004). Beyond the individual: The impact of ethnic context and classroom behavioral norms on victims' adjustment. *Developmental Psychology, 40,* 1159–1172.

Bennett, G.G., Wolin, K.Y., Robinson E.L., Fowler, S., & Edwards C.L. (2005). Perceived racial/ethnic harassment and tobacco use among African American young adults. *American Journal of Public Health, 95,* 238–240.

Bernal, M.E., Knight, G.P., Garza, C.A., Ocampo, K.A., & Cota, M.K. (1990). The development of ethnic identity in Mexican-American children. *Hispanic Journal of Behavioral Sciences, 12*, 3–24.

Berry, J.W., Phinney, J.S., Sam, D., & Vedder, P. (Eds.)(2006a). *Immigrant youth in cultural transition: Acculturation, identity and adaptation across national contexts.* Mahwah, NJ: Lawrence Erlbaum Associates.

Berry, J., Phinney, J., Sam, D., & Vedder, P. (2006b). Immigrant youth: Acculturation, identity and adaptation. *Applied Psychology: An International Review, 55*, 303–332.

Bourhis, R.Y., Moise, L.C., Perreault, S., & Senecal, S. (1997). Towards an interactive acculturation model: A social psychological approach. *International Journal of Psychology, 32*, 369–386.

Bowen-Reid, T.L., & Harrell, J.P. (2002). Racist experiences and health outcomes: an examination of spirituality as a buffer. *Journal of Black Psychology, 28*, 18–36.

Branscombe, N.R., Schmitt, M.T., & Harvey, R. (1999). Perceiving pervasive discrimination among African Americans: Implications for group identification and well-being. *Journal of Personality and Social Psychology, 77*, 135–149.

Brondolo, E., ver Halen, N.B., Pencille, M., Beatty, D., & Contrada, R.J. (2009). Coping with racism: A selective review of the literature and a theoretical and methodological critique. *Journal of Behavioral Medicine, 32*, 64–88.

Brown, T.N., Williams, D.R., Jackson, J.S., Neighbors, H.W., Torres, M., Sellers S.L., & Brown, K.T. (2000). Being black and feeling blue: the mental health consequences of racial discrimination. *Race and Society, 2*, 117–131.

Caldwell, C.H., Kohn-Wood, L.P., Schmeelk-Cone, K.H., Chavous, T.M., & Zimmerman, M.A. (2004). Racial discrimination and racial identity as risk or protective factors for violent behaviors in African American young adults. *American Journal of Community Psychology, 33*, 91–105.

Clark, R., & Gochett, P. (2006). Interactive effects of perceived racism and coping responses predict a school-based assessment of blood pressure in Black youth. *Annals of Behavioral Medicine, 32*, 1–9.

Cohen, G.L., & Garcia, J. (2005). 'I am us': Negative stereotypes as collective threats. *Journal of Personality and Social Psychology, 89*, 566–582.

Denscombe, M., Szulc, H., Patrick, C., & Wood, A. (1986). Ethnicity and friendship: the contrast between sociometric research and fieldwork observation in primary school classrooms. *British Educational Research Journal, 12*, 221–236.

Dovidio, J.F., Gaertner, S.L., & Kawakami, K. (2003). Intergroup contact: The past and the future. *Group Processes and Intergroup Relations, 6*, 5–21.

Equal Opportunity Commission of the Government of South Australia (2010). *What is discrimination?* Retrieved on April 26th, 2011, from http://www.eoc.sa.gov.au/eo-you/what-discrimination.

Finch, B.K., Kolody, B., & Vega, W.A. (2000). Perceived discrimination and depression among Mexican-origin adults in California. *Journal of Health and Social Behavior, 41*, 295–313.

Foster, G. (2008). Names will never hurt me: Racially distinct names and identity in the undergraduate classroom. *Social Science Research, 37*, 934–952.

Fuligni, A.J. (1998). The adjustment of children from immigrant families. *Current Directions in Psychological Science, 7*, 99–103.

Gaertner, S.L., & Dovidio, J.F. (2000). *Reducing intergroup bias: The Common Ingroup Identity Model.* Philadelphia: Psychology Press.

Garcia Coll, C., Lamberty, G., Jenkins, R., McAdoo, H.P., Crnic, K., Wasik, B.H., & Vazquez Garcia, H. (1996). An integrative model for the study of developmental competencies in minority children. *Child Development, 67*, 1891–1914.

Garcia Coll, C., & Marks, A. (2009). *Immigrant stories: Ethnicity and academics in middle childhood.* New York: Oxford University Press.

Garcia Coll, C., & Marks, A. (Eds.) (in press). *Is becoming American a developmental risk?* Washington: American Psychological Association.

Gaunt, R. (2009). Superordinate categorization as a moderator of mutual infrahumanization. *Group Processes & Intergroup Relations, 12*, 731–746.

Gee, G.C., Spencer, M.S., Chen, J., & Takeuchi, D. (2007). A nationwide study of discrimination and chronic health conditions among Asian Americans. *American Journal of Public Health, 97*, 1275–1282.

Gonzalez, K.V., Verkuyten, M., Weesie, J., & Poppe, E. (2008). Prejudice towards muslims in the Netherlands: Testing integrated threat theory. *British Journal of Social Psychology, 47*, 667–685.

Graham, J.A., & Cohen, R. (1997). Race and sex as factors in children's sociometric ratings and friendship choices. *Social Development, 6*, 355–372.

Harris, R., Tobias, M., Jeffreys, M., Waldegrave, K., Karlsen, S., & Nazroo, J. (2006). Racism and health: The relationship between experience of racial discrimination and health in New Zealand. *Social Science and Medicine, 63*, 1428–1441.

Heath, A.F., Rothon, C., & Kilpi, E. (2008). The second-generation in Western Europe: Education, unemployment, and occupational attainment. *Annual Review of Sociology, 34*, 211–235.

Holmes, R.M. (1995). *How young children perceive race.* Thousand Oaks, CA: Sage Publications.

Horenczyk, G., & Tatar, M. (1998). Friendship expectations among immigrant adolescents and their host peers. *Journal of Adolescence, 21*, 69–82.

Hughes, D., Witherspoon, D., Rivas-Drake, D., & West-Bey, N. (2009). Received ethnic/racial socialization messages and youth's academic and behavioral outcomes: examining the mediating role of ethnic identity and self esteem. *Cultural Diversity and Ethnic Minority Psychology, 15*, 112–124.

Jasinskaja-Lahti, I., & Liebkind, K. (2001). Perceived discrimination and psychological adjustment among Russian-speaking immigrant adolescents in Finland. *International Journal of Psychology, 36*, 174–185.

Jasinskaja-Lahti, I., Liebkind, K., Jaakkola, M., & Reuter, A. (2006). Perceived discrimination, social support networks, and psychological well-being among three immigrant groups. *Journal of Cross-cultural Psychology, 37*, 293–311.

Kao, G., & Joyner, K. (2004). Does race and ethnicity matter between friends? Activities among interracial, interethnic, and intraethnic adolescent friends. *Sociological Quarterly, 45*, 557–573.

Kao, G., & Vaquera, E. (2006). The salience of racial and ethnic identification in friendship choices among Hispanic adolescents. *The Hispanic Journal of Behavioral Sciences, 28*, 23–47.

Karlsen, S., & Nazroo, N.Y. (2002). Relation between racial discrimination, social class, and health among ethnic minority groups. *American Journal of Public Health, 92*, 624–631.

Knight, G.P., Bernal, M.E., Garza, C.A., Cota, M.K., & Ocampo, K.A. (1993). Family socialization and the ethnic identity of Mexican-American children. *Journal of Cross-Cultural Psychology, 24*, 99–114.

Kochenderfer-Ladd, B., & Pelletier, M. (2008). Teachers' views and beliefs about bullying: Influences on classroom management strategies and students' coping with peer victimization. *Journal of School Psychology, 46*, 431–453.

Krieger, N., & Sidney, S. (1996). Racial discrimination and blood pressure: The CARDIA Study of Young Black and White Adults. *American Journal of Public Health, 86*, 1370–1378.

Kromhout, M., & Vedder, P. (1996). Cultural inversion in children from the Antilles and Aruba in the Netherlands. *Anthropology and Education Quarterly, 27*, 568–586.

Lee, S.J. (1994). Behind the model-minority stereotype: Voices and high- and low-achieving Asian American students. *Anthropology & Education Quarterly, 25*, 413–429.

Liebkind, K. (2006). Ethnic identity and acculturation. In D.L. Sam & J.W. Berry (Eds.), *The Cambridge handbook of acculturation psychology* (pp. 78–96). Cambridge,: Cambridge University Press.

Liebkind, K., & Jasinskaja-Lahti, I. (2000). The influence of experiences of discrimination on psychological stress: A comparison of seven immigrant groups. *Journal of Community & Applied Social Psychology, 10*, 1–16.

Liebkind, K., Jasinskaja-Lahti, I., & Solheim, E. (2004). Cultural identity, perceived discrimination, and parental support as determinants of immigrants school adjustments: Vietnamese youth in Finland. *Journal of Adolescent Research, 19*, 635–656.

Lowell, B., & Gerova, S. (2004). Immigrants and the healthcare workforce – Profiles and shortages. *Work and Occupations, 31*, 474–498.

Mac an Ghaill, M. (1989). Coming-of-age in 1980s England: reconceptualising black students' schooling experience. *British Journal of Sociology of Education, 10*, 273–286.

Marks, A.K., Szalacha, L.S., Boyd, H.J., & Garcia Coll, C. (2007). Emerging ethic identity and interethnic social preferences in middle childhood. Findings from the Children of Immigrants Development in Context (CIDC) study. *International Journal of Behavioral Development 31(5)*, 501–513.

Masson, C.N., & Verkuyten, M. (1993). Prejudice, ethnic identity, contact and ethnic group preferences among Dutch young adolescents. *Journal of Applied Social Psychology, 23*, 156–168.

May, P. (1994). *Making multicultural education work*. Clevedon: Multilingual Matters.

McNeilly, M.D., Robinson, E.L., Anderson, N.B., Pieper, C.F., Shah, A., Toth, P.S., Martin, P., Jackson, D., Saulter, T.D., White, C., Kuchibatla, M., Collado, S.M., & Gerin, W. (1995). Effects of racist provocation and social support on cardiovascular reactivity in African American women. *International Journal of Behavioral Medicine, 2*, 321–338.

McPherson, M., Smith-Lovin, L., & Cook, J. (2001). Birds of a feather: Homophily in social networks. *Annual Review of Sociology, 27*, 415—444.

Merritt, M.M., Benett, G.G., Jr., Williams, R.B., Edwards, C.L., & Soller, J.J., III. (2006). Perceived racism and cardiovascular reactivity and recovery to personally relevant stress. *Health Psychology, 25*, 364–369.

Milner, D. (1983). *Children and race: Ten years on*. London: Ward Lock.

Modood, T. (2004). Capitals, ethnic identity and educational qualifications. *Cultural Trends, 13*, 87–105.

Mooney, A., Creeser, R., & Blatchford, P. (1991). Children's view on teasing and fighting in junior schools. *Educational Research, 33*:103–112.

Mossakowski, K. (2003). Coping with perceived discrimination: Does ethnic identity protect mental health? *Journal of Health and Social Behavior 44*, 318–331.

Mustillo, S., Krieger, N., Gunderson, E.P., Sidney, S., McCreath, H., & Kiefe, C.I. (2004). Self-reported experiences of racial discrimination and Black–White differences in preterm and low-birth weight deliveries: The CARDIA Study. *American Journal of Public Health, 94*, 2125–2131.

Noh, S., Beiser, M., Kaspar, V., Hou, F., & Rummens, J. (1999). Perceived racial discrimination, depression and coping. *Journal of Health and Social Behavior, 40*, 193–207.

Noh, S., & Kaspar, V. (2003). Perceived discrimination and depression: moderating effects of coping, acculturation, and ethnic support. *American Journal of Public Health, 93*, 232–238.

Ogbu, J.U., & Simons, H.D. (1998). Voluntary and involuntary minorities: A culturale-cological theory of school performance with some implications for education. *Anthropology and Education Quarterly, 29*, 155–188.

Olweus, D. (1993). *Bullying at school. What we know and what we can do.* Oxford: Blackwell.

Olweus, D. (1997). Bully/victim problems in school: Facts and intervention. *European Journal of Psychology of Education, 12*, 495–510.

Oortwijn, M., Boekaerts, M., Vedder, P., & Fortuin, J. (2008). The impact of a cooperative learning experience on pupils' popularity, non-cooperativeness, and ethnic bias in multiethnic elementary schools. *Educational Psychology, 28*, 211–221.

Ouarasse, O.A. & van de Vijver, F.J.R. (2005). The role of demographic variables and acculturation attitudes in predicting sociocultural and psychological adaptation in Moroccans in the Netherlands. *International Journal of Intercultural Relations, 29*, 251–272.

Pachter, L.M., & Garcia Coll, C. (2009). Racism and Child Health: A Review of the Literature and Future Directions. *Journal of Developmental and Behavioral Pediatrics, 30*, 255–263.

Paradies, Y. (2006). A systematic review of empirical research on self-reported racism and health. *International Journal of Epidemiology, 35*, 888–901.

Parekh, B. (2002). *Rethinking multiculturalism: Cultural diversity and political theory*. London: MacMillan.

Pascoe, E.A., & Richman, L.S. (2009). Perceived discrimination and health: A meta-analytic review. *Psychological Bulletin, 135,* 531–554.

Pettigrew, T.F. (1998). Intergroup contact theory. *Annual Review of Psychology, 49,* 65–85.

Pettigrew, T.F., & Tropp, L.R. (2006). A meta-analytic test of intergroup contact theory. *Journal of Personality and Social Psychology, 90,* 751–783.

Phalet, K., & Schönpflug, U. (2001). Intergenerational transmission of collectivism and achievement values in two acculturation contexts: The case of Turkish families in Germany and Turkish and Moroccan families in the Netherlands. *The Journal of Cross-Cultural Psychology, 32,* 186–201.

Phinney, J. (1989). Stages of ethnic identity development in minority group adolescents. *Journal of Early Adolescence, 9,* 34–49.

Phinney, J., Horenczyk, G., Liebkind, K., & Vedder, P. (2001). Ethnic identity, immigration, and well-being: an interactional perspective. *Journal of Social Issues, 57,* 493–510.

Phinney, J.S., & Kohatsu, E.L. (1997). Ethnic and racial identity development and mental health. In J. Schulenberg, J.L. Maggs & K. Hurrelmann (Eds.), *Health risks and developmental transitions during adolescence* (pp. 420–443). New York: Cambridge University Press.

Phinney, J.S., Romero, I., Nava, M., & Huang, D. (2001). The role of language, parents, and peers in ethnic identity among adolescents in immigrant families. *Journal of Youth and Adolescence, 30,* 135–153.

Portes, A., & Zhou, M. (1993). The new second generation: Segmented assimilation and its variants. *Annals of the American Academy of Political & Social Science, 530,* 74–96.

Psaty, B.M., Furberg, C.D., Kuller, L.H., Cushman, M., Savage, P.J., Levine, D., et al. (2001). Association between blood pressure level and the risk of myocardial infarction, stroke, and total mortality. *Archives of Internal Medicine, 161,* 1183–1192.

Quintana, S.M., Castañeda-English, P., & Ybarra, V.C. (1999). Role of perspective-taking ability and ethnic socialization in the development of adolescent ethnic identity. *Journal of Research on Adolescence, 9,* 161–184.

Reynolds, T. (2007). Friendship networks, social capital and ethnic identity: Researching the perspectives of Caribbean young people in Britain. *Journal of Youth Studies, 10,* 383–398.

Richeson, J.A., & Nussbaum, R.J. (2004). The impact of multiculturalism versus color-blindness on racial bias. *Journal of Experimental Social Psychology, 40,* 417–423.

Rigby, K. (2008). *Children and Bullying: How parents and educators can reduce bullying at school.* Oxford: Blackwell Publishing.

Rodriguez, J., Umaña-Taylor, A., Smith, E., & Johnson, D. (2009). Cultural processes in parenting and youth outcomes: Examining a model of racial-ethnic socialization and identity in diverse populations. *Cultural Diversity and Ethnic Minority Psychology, 15,* 106–111.

Rosenbloom, S.R., & Way, N. (2004). Experiences of discrimination among African American, Asian American, and Latino adolescents in an urban high school. *Youth and Society, 35,* 420–451.

Ryan, R.M., & Deci, E.L. (2000). Self-determination theory and the facilitation of intrinsic motivation, social development, and well being. *American Psychologist, 55,* 68–78.

Sellers, R.M., Caldwell, C.H., Schmeelk-Cone, K.H., & Zimmerman, M.A. (2003). Racial identity, Racial discrimination, perceived stress, and psychological distress among African American young adults. *Journal of Health and Social Behavior, 44,* 302–317.

Sherif, M. (1966). *In common predicament: Social psychology of intergroup conflict and cooperation.* Boston: Houghton-Mifflin.

Stevens, P. (2007). Researching race/ethnicity and educational inequality in English secondary schools: A critical review of the research literature between 1980 and 2005, *Review of Educational Research, 77,* 147–185.

Stevens, P., Clycq, N., Timmerman, Ch., & Van Houtte, M. (2011). Researching race/ethnicity and educational inequality in the Netherlands: A critical review of the research literature between 1980 and 2008'. *British Educational Research Journal, 37,* 5–43.

Stevens, G., Pels, T., Bengi-Arslan, L., Verhulst, F.C., Vollebergh, W.A.M., & Crijnen, A.A.M. (2003). Parent, teacher and self-reported problem behavior in the Netherlands: Comparing Moroccan immigrant with Dutch and with Turkish immigrant children and adolescents. *Social Psychiatry and Psychiatric Epidemiology, 38,* 576–585.

Suárez-Orozco, M.M. (2001). Globalization, immigration, and education: The research agenda. *Harvard Education Review, 71,* 345–365.

Tajfel, H., & Turner, J.C. (1986). The social identity theory of intergroup behavior. In S. Worchel & W. Austin (Eds.), *Psychology of intergroup relationsIntergroup Relations* (pp. 7–24). Chicago: Nelson-Hall.

Tatar, M., & Horenczyk, G. (2003). Diversity-related burnout among teachers. *Teaching and Teacher Education, 19,* 397–408.

Tatum, B.D. (2003). *Why are all the black kids sitting together in the cafeteria?* New York: Basic Books.

Tenenbaum, H.R., & Ruck, M.D. (2007). Are teachers'expectations different for racial minority than for European American students? A meta-analysis. *Journal of Educational Psychology, 99,* 253–273.

Thornton, M.C., Chatters, L.M., Taylor, R.J., & Allen, W.R. (1990). Sociodemographic and environmental correlates of racial socialization by Black parents. *Child Development, 61,* 401–409.

Titzmann, P.F., Silbereisen, R.K., & Schmitt-Rodermund, E. (2007). Friendship homophily among diaspora migrant adolescents in Germany and Israel. *European Psychologist, 12,* 181–195.

Van Geel, M., & Vedder, P. (2009). Perceived discrimination and psychological adjustment of immigrants. A review of research. In I. Jasinskaja-Lahti & T. Anna Mähönen (Eds.), *Identities, intergroup relations and acculturation: the cornerstone of intercultural encounters* (pp. 179–190). Helsinki: Gaudeamus Helsinki University Press.

Van Geel, M., & Vedder, P. (2011). The role of family obligations and school adjustment in explaining the immigrant paradox. *Journal of Youth and Adolescence, 40,* 187–196.

Vedder, P. (2006). Black and white schools in the Netherlands. *European Education, 38,* 36–49.

Vedder, P., Berry, J., Sabatier, C., & Sam, D. (2009). The intergenerational transmission of values in national and immigrant families: The role of zeitgeist. *Journal of Youth and Adolescence, 38*, 642–653.

Vedder, P., Bouwer, E., & Pels, T. (1996). *Multicultural child care*. Clevedon: Multilingual Matters.

Vedder, P., & Horenczyk, G. (2006). Acculturation and the school context. In D.L. Sam & J.W. Berry (Eds.), *Psychology of acculturation; international perspectives* (pp. 419–438). Cambridge: Cambridge University Press

Vedder, P., Horenczyk, G., & Liebkind, K. (2006). Problems in ethno-cultural diverse educational settings and strategies to cope with these challenges. *Educational Research Review, 1*, 157–168.

Vedder, P., & Phinney, J.S. (in press). Identity formation in bicultural youth: A developmental perspective. In Veronica Benet-Martinez & Ying-yi Hong (Eds.), *The Oxford handbook of multicultural identity*. New York: Oxford University Press.

Verkuyten, M. (1998). Perceived discrimination and self-esteem among ethnic minority adolescents. *Journal of Social Psychology, 138*, 479–493.

Verkuyten, M., & Thijs, J. (2002). Racist victimization among children in the Netherlands: the effects of ethnic group and school. *Ethnic and Racial Studies, 25*, 310–331.

Vollmer G. (2000). Praise and stigma: teachers' constructions of the 'typical ESL student'. *Journal of Intercultural Studies, 21*, 53–66.

Wagenaar, W., & van Donselaar, J. (2008). Racistisch en extreemrechts geweld in 2007. In J. van Donselaar & P.R. Rodrigues (Red.). *Monitor Racisme & Extremisme. Achtste Rapportage* (pp. 16–41). Amsterdam: Anne Frank Stichting/Amsterdam University Press.

Williams, D.R., & Mohammed, S. (2009). Discrimination and racial disparities in health: evidence and needed research. *Journal of Behavioral Medicine 32*, 20–47.

Yen, I.H., Ragland, D.R., Greiner, B.A., & Fisher, J.M. (1999). Racial discrimination and alcohol-related behavior in urban transit operators: Findings from the San Francisco Muni health and safety study. *Public Health Reports, 114*, 448–458.

Zentella, A.C. (Ed.) (2005). *Building on strength: Language and literacy in Latino families and communities*. New York: Teachers College Press.

Paul Vedder
Department of Education and Child Studies, Leiden University
PO Box 9555
NL–2300 RB Leiden (The Netherlands)
E-Mail VEDDER@FSW.leidenuniv.nl

# Immigrant Family Separations: The Experience of Separated, Unaccompanied, and Reunited Youth and Families

Carola Suárez-Orozco · María G. Hernández

New York University, New York, N.Y., USA

## Abstract

Migration is transforming the shape of the family. Worldwide, more than 214 million are immigrants or refugees, and in the US about 12% of the population are foreign-born with more than a fifth of the nation's children growing up in immigrant homes. During the course of migration, many families must make the painful decision to leave behind loved ones in their home countries, including children, spouses, parents and extended family members. Sociologists and clinical psychologists have documented the unfavorable psychosocial consequences associated with family separations, though we have not fully understood how strategies employed by families shape youths' overall well-being from a developmental perspective. To fill this gap, we utilized qualitative data from two large studies to provide insight into the experiences of separated-reunited youth and their families, and separated unaccompanied minors. Our findings revealed that the separated-reunited and unaccompanied minors experienced strain in their family relationships during the separation, and attempted to alleviate their angst by maintaining contact through numerous channels. Although separated-reunited families are confronted with reestablishing relationships that were tarnished due to the separation, through remarkable strengths, resources, determination and resilience they readjusted. Unlike separated-reunited youth, unaccompanied minors encountered the pressures of taking on adult-like responsibilities, such as parenting themselves, working to financially support themselves, at times their family members in their countries of origin, and attending school full-time. We discuss the implications that migration-related separations have for the psychological and academic adjustment of youth, development, and policy.

Copyright © 2012 S. Karger AG, Basel

Worldwide, more than two hundred and fourteen million are immigrants and refugees. In the US today, about 12% of the population are foreign-born [US Census Bureau, 2000] and more than a fifth of the nation's children are growing up in immigrant homes [Rong & Preissle, 1998]. During the course of migration, many families must make the painful decision to leave behind loved ones in their home countries, including children, spouses, parents and extended family members [United Nations Development Programme, UNDP, 2009]. Thus, migration and forces of globalization are transforming the shape of the family [UNDP, 2009].

Increasingly, the experience of transnational families can be characterized by 'separation and reunification of different members of the family unit over time' [Tyyska, 2007, p. 91]. When families separate, they often expect to reunite soon. However, in the process of migration, families often endure prolonged periods of separation before they are reunited again [Suárez-Orozco, Todorova & Louie, 2002]. The actual manifestations of family separation and reunification processes vary widely depending on the purpose of the migration and social and cultural-specific contexts of the families. 'Stepwise' or 'serial' fashion migration is a common strategy for immigrant families [Hondagneu-Sotelo, 1992; Orellana, Thorne, Chee & Lam, 2001]. Historically, the pattern was of the father going ahead, establishing himself while sending remittances home, and then bringing the wife and children as soon as it was financially possible. Today, the first world's demand for service workers draw mothers from a variety of developing countries to care for 'other people's children' [Gratton, 2007; Hondagneu-Sotelo, 2003; Hondagneu-Sotelo & Avila, 1997]. In cases where mothers initiate the migrations, they leave their children in the care of extended family such as grandparents or aunts along with the father if he is still part of the family. In many other cases, both parents go ahead, leaving the children in the care of extended family [Bernhard, Landolt & Goldring, 2006; Qin & Albin, 2010; Scalabrini Migration Center, 2003], while in a more recent documented trend adolescent children lead in immigration as 'unaccompanied minors', without any parents [Hernández, 2009; Martínez, 2009; Wexler Love, 2010]. These adolescents typically emigrate from Latin American countries, such as Mexico, Honduras, and Nicaragua seeking employment or educational opportunities [Hernández, 2009; Martínez, 2009; Wexler Love, 2010]. Upper-middle-class families from East Asian countries such as Hong Kong, Korea, and Taiwan send middle- and high-school-aged students to study abroad as 'astronaut kids', living with the mother while the father remains in the homeland [Ong, 1999; Waters, 2002] or as 'parachute kids', living with extended or fictive kin while both parents remain in the homeland [Ong, 1999; Zhou, 2009]. Another long-documented practice is that of children being sent back to the homeland to be taken care of by grandparents. Typically, unruly adolescents have been sent back to be resocialized by their grandparents [Foner, 2009; Smith, 2006], but increasingly, infants and toddlers are being sent back to be cared for by extended family while parents work [Bohr, Whitfield & Chan, 2009; Gaytán, Xue & Yoshikawa, 2006]. In recent years, families with undocumented parents have involuntarily been wrenched apart by workplace as well as in-home raids conducted by immigration authorities [Capps, Castañeda, Chaudry & Santos, 2007; Chaudry, Pedroza, Castañeda, Santos & Scott, 2010].

Reunification of the entire family can often take many years, especially when complicated by financial hurdles as well as immigration laws [Bernhard et al., 2006; Menjívar & Abrego, 2009]. When it is time for the children to arrive, they may be brought to the new land all together or one at a time [Bernhard et al., 2006]. Though parents maintain contact during the separation period through letters, phone calls, personal visits, and contributions to the material well-being of their children, these separation-reunification processes involve difficult psychological experiences for the children during the separation as well as after the reunification [Suárez-Orozco et al., 2002]. For the children, these serial migrations result in two sets of disruptions in attachments – first from the parent, and then from the caretaker to whom the child has become attached during the parent-child separation [Ambert & Krull, 2006; Bernhard et al., 2006; Wong, 2006].

This practice of 'familyhood' even across the national borders' [Bryceson & Vuorela, 2002, p. 3] has been well documented by sociologists [Dreby, 2007, 2009; Foner, 2009; Glick-Schiller & Fouron, 1992; Hondagneu-Sotelo, 2003] and economists [Abrego, 2009; Suro, 2003], but has largely failed to be noted in the developmental literature. In particular, the children's perspectives on the separation experience and its developmental implications have been overlooked until recently [Suárez-Orozco, Bang & Kim, 2011]. This chapter first aims to summarize the current knowledge of transnational separations and reunifications through a review of existing literature, including studies related to separated-reunited families, unaccompanied minors, and parachute kids[1]. Then, through qualitative analyses of data from the Longitudinal Immigrant Student Adaptation (LISA) study [Suárez-Orozco, Suárez-Orozco & Todorova, 2008] and the Immigrant Central American and Mexican Adolescent (ICAMA) study [Hernández, 2009], the authors share insights into immigrant families' subjective experiences of the separation-reunification process.

**Prevalence of Separations of Transnational Familyhood**

Despite the commonality of family separations during the migration process, prevalence and cross-cultural patterns of immigrant family separations is largely unknown, and the estimates from available studies vary widely. Among the participants of the LISA study – a study of 385 adolescent newcomers from China, Mexico, the Dominican Republic, Haiti, and Central America, approximately one third of the participants reported experiencing a separation from at least one parent [Suárez-Orozco et al., 2011]. Significant differences between ethnic groups were observed with regard to family separation: Chinese families were the least likely to be separated over the course of migration (52%), while the vast majority of Central American (88%) and Haitian children (85%) were separated from either or both of their parents during the course of migration. Approximately 26% of children in the sample were separated from both parents, a pattern most often occurring in Central American families (54%). In cases where the child was separated from only one parent, about 26% of children were separated from the mother, while about 20% of children were separated from the father. Separations from mothers occurred most frequently among Dominican (40%) families, and separations from fathers were most frequently found among Mexican (33%) families. Of the participants who were separated only from their mothers, 44% of Central American children endured separations lasting 4 or more years as did approximately a quarter of both the Dominican and Haitian families. Chinese and Mexican children underwent fewer and shorter separations from their mothers. When separation from the father occurred during migration, it was often a very lengthy or permanent one. For those families who were separated, 28% had separations from fathers that lasted over 4 years. This was the case for 45% of the Haitian, 41% of Central American, and 27% of the Dominican families.

In a more recent study conducted in Montreal, a similar pattern of separation was found [Rousseau et al., 2009]. Among 254 first- and second-generation immigrant origin high school students from the Philippines and the Caribbean, approximately 62% of the Filipino origin participants and 38% of the Caribbean origin participants had experienced separations. It is important to note that this study did not disaggregate by generation. Since separations are unlikely to occur in the second generation, this is a low estimate of what the separation rates would be for a first-generation sample.

In a US nationally representative survey (n = 1,772) that restricted its sample to documented immigrants (in contrast to the two studies noted above which included unauthorized immigrants), nearly a third of the participants between ages 6 and 18 had been separated from at least one parent for 2 or more years. Notably, the rates of separation were highest for children of Latin American origin than of Asia and other parts of the world [Gindling & Poggio, 2009]. Thus, in keeping with reports in other post-industrial settings (UNDP,

---

[1] We briefly extrapolate from the literature on parachute kids to raise important empirical and practical issues about how separation from parents and immigrating alone as an adolescent affects the development of immigrant youths, their relationships with their parents and families, and their experiences of adaptation in the host country. We fully recognize that the purpose of immigration of parachute kids is distinct from unaccompanied minors. Parachute kids enter the US as authorized visa holders, and the financial resources they receive from their parents in the homeland allow them to live a comfortable life in the US.

2009), separations from biological parents appear to be quite frequent among first-generation immigrants in North America.

Regrettably, little is known about the immigration prevalence rates of unaccompanied minors. Data that do exist come from a few qualitative studies [Hernández, 2009; Martínez, 2009; Wexler Love, 2010] and statistics maintained on apprehended youth by the Office of Refugee Resettlement in the Division of Unaccompanied Children Services, under the Administration of Children and Families. Regarding studies with samples of unaccompanied minors, Hernández [2009] found that out of 30 participants, 27% were unaccompanied minors, while in the study by Martínez [2009] 3 out of 7 participants were unaccompanied minors, and 6 out of 10 of Wexler Love [2010] participants were considered unaccompanied. In 2009, 6,074 unaccompanied children were apprehended [US Department of Health and Human Services, 2009]. The Division of Unaccompanied Children Services consider unaccompanied children to be those who: have no lawful immigration status in the US, have not attained 18 years of age, and with respect to whom: (a) there is no parent or legal guardian in the US or (b) no parent or legal guardian in the US is available to provide care and physical custody. Nevertheless, these data fail to provide an adequate representation of the number of adolescent children who lead in immigration, without their parents, because it only represents those that have come to the attention of immigration services.

## Youth's Experience of Family Separations and Reunifications

In this section, we present findings from sociological, clinical, and developmental literature regarding the impact of separations and reunifications on family relations and psychological experience, and its implication in academic development in the host countries for families experiencing 'stepwise' immigration and 'unaccompanied minors'.

### Changes in Family Relations

While the discipline of developmental psychology has been slow to realize the number of children and youth caught up in transnational family constellations, sociologists and clinical psychologists have been documenting this phenomenon over the last decade or so.

From the sociological data, several patterns emerge. The clearest evidence points to the disruption to family relations. In broad strokes, this research – based largely on transnational studies conducted on Central American and Mexican families during the separation phase in the country of origin and during the reunification stage in the receiving country – reveal some fairly consistent insights [Foner, 2009]. During the separations phase, children appear to adjust more easily to the father being away, perhaps because this is consistent with gender expectations and patterns of childrearing [Dreby, 2007]. However, when the mother or both parents are away, the children often attach to the substitute caretaker. Mothers (more so than fathers) often maintain regular contact with their children [Abrego, 2009; Dreby, 2009] attempting to maintain 'emotional intimacy from a distance' [Dreby, 2009, p. 34]. Younger children often begin to emotionally withdraw from their mothers, and adolescents typically become either quite independent or act out aggressively [Dreby, 2009; Smith, 2006]. Similarly, the maintenance of close relationships is also challenging for unaccompanied minors and parachute kids. For instance, Hernández [2009] findings suggest that for unaccompanied minors, the relationships they have with parents become estranged and distant because of the lack of daily sharing that used to occur in the homeland with family members prior to immigration. Zhou [1998] findings in her study of parachute kids also underscore the estrangement that these adolescents endure when separated from their parents. Parachute kids and their parents maintain contact through phone calls and yearly visits, but these do not suffice over time to maintain the fullness of the relationship prior to separation. Over time, parents develop guilt and consequently become more easygoing with their children, while the children have gotten used to living by themselves and have become more independent. To comfort themselves about their separation, they overcompensate by understanding that education takes priority, and associate the physical separation as a sign of caring. Thus, for both 'stepwise' migrated, unaccompanied children, and parachute kids maintaining long-distance emotional intimacy with parents over an extended physical absence is challenging.

During the reunification stage for 'stepwise' migrated families, children and youth often report ambivalence about leaving behind their beloved extended family caregivers and friends and are anxious about meeting members of the biological family, including parents, who have become strangers over the prolonged separation [Foner, 2009; Menjívar & Abrego, 2009]. Parents often report struggles with asserting their authority and frustration that their financial and emotional sacrifices are not fully appreciated by their children [Abrego, 2009; Dreby, 2006; Foner, 2009; Menjívar & Abrego, 2009; Zhou, 2009].

There is also a body of literature derived from clinical reports, which points to a pattern of family conflict during the family reunification phase [Glasgow & Gouse-Shees, 1995; Sciarra, 1999]. This literature suggests that over time, the substitute family system for the child left behind may have evolved in such a way that it excludes the parent who has been away, making reunification of the family system difficult [Falicov, 2007; Partida, 1996]. Parents tend to expect their children to be grateful for their sacrifices, but often find that their children are ambivalent about joining their parents in the migratory process [Boti & Bautista, 1999; Rousseau et al., 2009; Sciarra, 1999]. Also, children may be disappointed for how their real parents turn out to be, compared to their fantasies and expectations about the life in the US. [Artico, 2003]. After the long separation period, youth left behind feel competitive with siblings born in the host country for the mother's affection [Arnold, 2006], and parents often report having difficulties in establishing functional intra-family relations [Arnold, 2006; Boti & Bautista, 1999; Sewell-Coker, Hamilton-Collins & Fein, 1985]. The longer the separation they undergo, the less likely adolescents report being able to identify with their parents or being willing to conform to their rules at the time of reunification [Smith, Lalonde & Johnson, 2004]. Reestablishing control and authority may be complicated by parental guilt, which may result in inconsistencies and overindulgence [Arnold, 1991; Burke, 1980]. A 'continual pattern of rejection and counter-rejection' may emerge, leading families to seek treatment [Glasgow & Gouse-Shees, 1995]. Thus, many reunified families experience tensions, conflict, and adjustment difficulties particularly during the phase of adolescent development [Crawford-Brown & Melrose, 2001; Lashley, 2000].

While the research from sociological and clinical perspective is useful, there is more to learn about the family separation phenomenon and its impact on immigrant youth's lives. Particularly, much of the richest sociological research on the phenomenon has been conducted only with mothers [e.g. Hondagneu-Sotelo & Avila, 1997; Levitt, 2001] or with single country samples [e.g. Dominicans-Levitt, 2001; Mexicans-Dreby, 2007, 2009; Salvadorans-Abrego, 2009]. The clinical literature does not shed adequate light on understanding the effects of separations on normally functioning families, as only those who are in need of treatment are represented. The data are generally focused on the complication in reunification rather than on the separation. Moreover, to date, these studies have largely been qualitative and have failed to also explore the experiences of children leading in migration (unaccompanied minors). Thus, while we have some insights into the effects of transnationalism on immigrant families [Falicov, 2007; Foner, 2009], we know little about normative developmental outcomes for immigrant youth from diverse backgrounds.

*Psychological Consequences*

Family contexts have been well established to have critical implications for the functioning of children and youth [Bronfenbrenner & Morris, 1998; Small & Covalt, 2006]. Disruptions in family systems are likely to have implications for the well-being of children. A number of clinical studies (conducted with Caribbean families in Canada and the UK, along with a few studies on Caribbean and Latino families in the US) show that there are substantial negative psychological repercussions for immigrant children and youth who have been separated from their parents [Smith et al., 2004; Suárez-Orozco et al., 2011]. These studies uniformly point to complications occurring both during the separation phase when the child is left with relatives and during the reunification phase when the child joins the parents. While apart from the parent, clinical studies report that children and youth may feel abandoned and may respond with despair and detachment [Artico, 2003]. Once reunified, they often miss those who have cared for them and with whom they have developed strong attachments in their parent's absence as well as extended family members and friends [Arnold, 1991; Sciarra, 1999]. Particularly when separations have been protracted, children and parents frequently report that they feel like strangers when they are reunited [Artico, 2003; Forman, 1993]. Attachment difficulties have been noted [Wilkes, 1992], and children and youth are often withdrawn from the parents with whom they are reunited [Burke, 1980; Suárez-Orozco et al., 2002] and report low self-esteem at the time of reunion [Smith et al., 2004]. Depressive responses have been noted in both children [Rutter, 1971] and mothers [Bernhard et al., 2006]. Children may have difficulty trusting others [Arnold, 2006; Artico, 2003], and those who experienced long-term separations are more likely to receive psychiatric services [Morgan et al., 2007]. Some youth may respond by externalizing, increased anger, and aggression [Burke, 1980; Dreby, 2007; Lashley, 2000; Smith, 2006; Wilkes, 1992]. Thus, previous research from sociological, clinical, and the limited developmental perspectives suggests that while children and youth may be the 'primary [intended] beneficiaries of their parents' sacrifice... [they] are often the last link to move abroad... [and] are left behind [to] pay the emotional price of separation from parents over the long run' [Dreby, 2007, p. 1051]. While these reports are important in delineating the syndrome and its clinical ramifications, they do not explain or help us better understand the consequences of separations of normally functioning families. These studies, because they are derived from clinical populations, focus only on families and youth who are unsuccessful in managing the separations without clinical intervention. This presents the possible danger of overly pathologizing the outcome of separations. Indeed, Rousseau et al. [2009] found that the experience of extended separation is associated with psychological symptoms and suggested that post-migration reorganization of the family and interaction with the host society may have greater influence on successes and difficulties of adaptation in the host countries than the migration-related family separation itself.

Similarly, in analyses of the LISA study, we found that children who were separated from their parents were more likely to report symptoms of anxiety and depression than those who were not separated in the initial years of immigration; however, 5 years later, these psychological symptoms seemed to have abated completely [Suárez-Orozco et al., 2011]. Youths who had undergone the longest separations from their mothers reported the highest levels of anxiety and depression. Generally, the highest levels of distress were reported by youths who underwent mid- and long-term separations.

*Implication in Academic Adaptation*

Early adolescence is a time of heightened risk for a 'downward educational spiral' [Eccles et al., 1993, p. 90], particularly when the educational environment does not meet developmental needs of youth. This is especially true to many newcomer immigrant youth who experienced separations from their parents during the migration process. Many of them grow up in nontraditional, complex household arrangements that include in some instances one parent remaining in the homeland [Hernández, Denton & McCartney, 2007; Suárez-Orozco et al., 2002] and going through emotionally painful separations and consequent complication in family relationships and psychological symptoms described above. A large proportion of immigrant-origin youth struggle to succeed in the educational system, performing poorly on a variety of academic indicators, including achievement tests, grades, dropout rates, and college attendance [Gándara & Contreras, 2010; Orfield & Lee, 2006]; evidence exists to suggest that family separation experience is one of the major factors contributing to their underachievement [Suárez-Orozco, Bang & Onaga, 2010; Suárez-Orozco et al., 2010b; Gindling & Poggio, 2008].

Academic underachievement is also a particular reality for unaccompanied minors who migrate in search of work. Many of these unaccompanied minors arrive to the US with particular beliefs about their life stages and their 'location in the transition to adulthood' [Martínez, 2009, p. 46], assuming full time employment and bypassing enrolling in school. However, for some unaccompanied minors once they find and settle into their job and learn about prospective educational opportunities, some will enroll in school. Nevertheless, these youth often have a difficult time managing their full-time employment demands with school responsibilities, which often leads to temporarily dropping out of school [Hernández, 2009].

Children separated from parents during migration are more likely to lag behind others their age in school and are more likely to drop out of high school [Gindling & Poggio, 2008]. Among Spanish-speaking immigrant youth, boys are particularly vulnerable to separation experience falling further behind their peers academically. It may be that the boys were more vulnerable to having fewer adults available to supervise them, though further research is required to unpack the reasons behind this pattern of outcome. Educational expectations are also lower among students separated from parents, especially for younger students [Wright, 2010].

The most alarming ramification of separations is its lasting influence on students' long-term academic trajectories. Recent analysis of the LISA study found that students who have experienced separation from their mothers were more likely to be precipitous decliners or slow decliners than high achievers. This was also the case for those separated from their fathers. Furthermore, the longer the separation from the father, the greater the negative effects were on academic trajectories [Suárez-Orozco et al., 2010a].

**Overview of the Studies**

Utilizing data from the LISA study [Suárez-Orozco et al., 2008] and the ICAMA study [Hernández, 2009], we present analyses of qualitative data gathered from parents and students from open-ended interview questions as well as ethnographic interviews to shed light on the separation and reunification experiences from the perspectives of immigrant youth and their parents. We will first describe the LISA study, followed by the ICAMA study.

*LISA Study*

Four hundred and seven immigrant youth participants (53% female) newly arrived from Central America, China, the Dominican Republic, Haiti, and Mexico were initially recruited from the Boston and San Francisco metropolitan areas. We negotiated entrance into school sites with high densities of immigrant students and enlisted the help of school authorities to identify youth who met the inclusion criteria: both parents must be from one of the five regions of origin, and students must have spent no more than a third of their lives in the US. Research assistants requested potential participants' involvement, assured them confidentiality, and obtained informed consent from parents.

Participants ranged in age from 9 to 14 at the beginning of the study (mean = 11.7 years of age), though Haitians on average were significantly younger by one year than the Dominicans and Chinese. All participants had been in the US less than a third of their lives (mean = 1.93 years). By year 5, the final sample included 309 students (Chinese = 72; Dominican = 60; Central American = 57; Haitian = 50; Mexican = 70) representing an attrition rate of 5% annually.

Students in the LISA study were recruited from over 50 schools in 7 districts representing typical contexts of reception for newcomer students from each of the groups of origin [US Census Bureau, 2000]. Because of normative developmental school transitions (from middle to high school) and high mobility of immigrant students, our participants transferred schools frequently over the course of the 5 years of the study. By the end of the study, they had had dispersed to nearly 125 schools; students' transfer rates ranged between 1 and 5 transfer incidents (mean = 2.4). Most of our students' schools were also highly racially and economically segregated. The schools they attended were characterized by high percentages of students living in poverty, with an average of 49.2% (SD = 23.5%) of students receiving free or reduced-cost lunch. The minority representation rate at the schools our students attended was, on average, 78.8% (SD = 23.2%) [see Suárez-Orozco et al., 2008 for detailed description of school contexts].

The study used a mixed-methods approach, which included school ethnographies, interview data collected over the course of 5 years from students, parents, and school personnel, as well as school records. Each year, students completed interviews either during or after school, depending upon the participant's availability and the activities occurring at school on the day of the interview. Bilingual RAs conducted all interviews orally on an individual basis in the participants' preferred language so as not to be affected by students' limited literacy skills. Each student interview took about 1.5–2 h to administer and involved a variety of question formats (open-ended, fill-in-the-blank, Likert scales, etc.). Parent interviews were conducted in their native languages the first and last years of the study at the participants' homes.

Teacher and administrative interviews were conducted both spontaneously during the course of ethnographic fieldwork as well as systematically across 20 school sites. We interviewed 75 teachers and administrators working in sites where we had 5 or more participating students. We selected a range of school qualities as well as teachers teaching across disciplines (math, language arts, English as a Second Language – ESL, science, social studies) with varying degrees of experience with immigrant students. The interview was designed to elicit both the strengths and the challenges faced of newcomer students. These semi-structured interviews typically lasted 1.5 hours, were tape recorded, and consisted of both open-ended and forced-choice items. Family separations spontaneously emerged as a particular challenge faced by immigrant students.

*Qualitative Data Sources*

The qualitative data presented here were gathered from several sources: (1) open-ended questions from the structured interviews conducted with the whole sample of the 407 informants originally recruited for the LISA study as well as their parents; (2) follow-up interviews focused on separation with 12 students who had undergone protracted separations, and (3) insights offered by school personnel in the course of our research in the schools collecting data.

*Open-Ended Questions.* In the first year of the study, parents were asked about their relationship with their child; and we found they often revealed information about their family separations and reunifications. Specifically, we asked: What kind of relationship did you have with your child before you came to the US? Has your relationship changed since you came to the US? In what ways? [If things have changed], what do you think are some of the reasons for these changes? After analyzing the first year data and realizing that such a large proportion of families had been separated during the course of migration, we added to the second year student interview several questions about the reunification process which were posed to all students who had been separated. These questions included: How did you feel when you were first reunited? Was there anything difficult or complicated about getting together? And how are things now?

*Follow-Up Separation Interviews.* During the second year of the LISA project, we selected 12 children who had undergone lengthy separations to participate in extended semi-structured 1.5- to 2-hour-long interviews focused on their experiences of separations and reunifications. These participants were selected to represent a range of types of separations, countries of origin, student genders, and patterns of separation (e.g. father only, mother only, and both, as well as varying lengths of separation). The interview explored the participants' experiences both during the separations as well as the reunifications phase.

*School Personnel Insights.* Lastly, we spent extensive time in schools over the course of our 5-year study and spoke to many teachers and administrators who knew we were studying immigrant student adaptation. Though we did not systematically interview school personnel about family separations, several spontaneously offered their thoughts about this issue as a problem they found that many immigrant students face.

## ICAMA Study

In the ICAMA study, 30 recently arrived adolescents from Central America and Mexico were recruited from four high schools in a mid-sized city in Wisconsin. The schools in which students were recruited from were over 60% majority White [see Hernández, 2009, for full school context descriptions]. School personnel who mainly worked with newcomer immigrant students helped identify students who were 14–20 years old at the time of recruitment, arrived in the US after 9 years old, and of Mexican or Central American origin. Participants also had to reside in the US from 3 months to 8 years. The wide range in age at arrival, and time residing in the US were used to sample a variety of ages and durations in the US in order to make comparisons between the adolescent ages and number of months and years in the US and duration and age of separation. The second author requested potential participants' involvement, assured them confidentiality, and obtained informed consent from parents or guardians.

Participants in the ICAMA study ranged in age from 14 to 19 at the beginning of the study (mean = 16.5). Participants recruited for this study ranged in their migration strategy, including 'stepwise' migrants, unaccompanied minors, and joint-parent migrations. The majority of participants (28) immigrated to the US between the ages of 12 and 17, with 2 participants arriving between the ages of 9 and 11. Ten participants reported having been in the US from 3 to 11 months, with 10 participants reporting being in the US between one year and 2 years, 11 months, and 10 participants said they have been in the US between 3 and 7 years.

Adolescents' age at separation varied among participants, with 14 adolescents experiencing separation between 6 and 10 years old, and 16 separating from their parents between 11 and 17 years old. Many reunited with their parent in their early and mid-adolescent years, with 3 who rejoined their parent between 9 and 12 years old. The length of parent-child separation also varied in this sample, with 16 being separated from their parents from 4 months to almost 4 years and 14 being separated for more than 5 years.

Unlike the LISA study with high-density immigrant schools, recently arrived immigrant students were a more recent phenomenon to this school district. As schools in this district observed an increase in the enrollment rate of immigrant Latino students, they adapted their services to meet the needs of this growing population by recruiting and hiring more Bilingual Resources Specialist, ESL teachers, and Bilingual Resource teachers. While many school districts nationally have abolished bilingual education programs, in particular where there are greater proportions of Latinos, this district still maintained a commitment to bilingual education. For recently arrived high school students, the district had a newcomer program that offered services for students who were new to the US and were at a beginning/preproduction level of English proficiency. Newcomer services provided students the English skills necessary to function in a new school, community, and country. Students participated in a newcomer class for a limited time and eventually moved to different types of ESL and/or bilingual support. There were a total of 24 ESL and bilingual teachers at the four high schools to support youth in acquiring English skills. Regardless of these efforts, at the high school level the curriculum mainly centered on implementing an ESL curriculum in content areas.

*Qualitative Data Sources*

The ICAMA study used three semi-structured interviews to explore how immigrant Latino youth adapted to and negotiated the demands of being in a new country, and how prior experiences in their country of origin shaped their US experiences. The follow-up interview took place 4–6 months after the initial interview, and the final interview was conducted a year after the initial interview.

Initial Interview

The interview aimed to learn from adolescents: (1) how they experienced separation and reunification from their parents; (2) how they adapted to US life, including how adolescents approached and coped with being in new contexts and how they understood their cultures of origin and US culture; (3) their ethnic identities; (4) their perceptions and experiences of discrimination; (5) their family relationships, and (6) the meanings they gave to psychological well being and when they felt happy, sad, and stressed. The interview asked similar questions of each participant, while tailoring follow-up questions and probes to each adolescent. Specific questions related to their separation experiences included: *Did* you and your family immigrate together or separately?; How did it affect you immigrating together or separately?; Why did you immigrate on different occasions; Even if your parents are in the USA or in your country of origin, tell me about the relationship you have with them; What has changed in the relationship with your parents since you moved to the USA?

Follow-Up Interview and Final Interview

The follow-up interview was used to confirm and build on each adolescent's prior interview by asking additional questions focusing on adolescent's adaptation to the US, his or her living conditions in the county of origin, perceived discrimination, his or her separation from family, and his or her future plans. After completing 5 initial interviews, it was evident that additional questions be generated for participants to clarify and elaborate on interview topics that had been addressed in the first interview.

The final interview asked participants similar questions as the initial interview to address their perceived changes in separation and reunification from their parents, their adaptation to US life, their ethnic identities, experiences of discrimination, their family relationships, and perceptions of their psychological well-being.

Coding of All Qualitative Data

Both the LISA and the ICAMA study employed an open-coding process using phrases and narratives as units of analysis [Strauss & Corbin, 1990]. During the first stage of the coding, emergent descriptive themes from all of the transcripts were identified. The initial set of independently identified themes was compared and integrated into a comprehensive list of coding categories [Miles & Huberman, 1994]. Once these 'pattern codes' [Miles & Huberman, 1994, p. 67] were identified, a second iteration of coding was conducted using another analytic procedure. First, we cross-referenced based on the kind of separations (mother only, father only, and both) and then by length of separations (short-term, medium-term, and long-term). Examination of the pattern codes and the types of separations revealed insights into the processes and meanings of the separations and reunifications for youth and their families. In the ICAMA study only, similar themes were collapsed and re-assigned one code. Any necessary recoding of interviews or adjustment to the coding scheme was completed at this stage. The criteria used to determine when categories and themes were significant were based on their frequency of appearance, proportional length, and vividness in the text [Lieblich, Tuval-Mashiach & Zibler, 1998].

In the LISA study only, the coders (who were not involved in the data collection process to guard against bias during the analytic and interpretative processes) refined the coding scheme 'by discussing the meanings of, and relationships between, each coding category, and identified rules for determining when a particular coding category should be assigned to a response' [Mattis et al., 2008, pp. 420–421]. Two coders assessed the reliability of the coding scheme using 10% percent of randomly selected narrative samples. The formula for inter-rater reliability was: inter-rater reliability = agreement/(agreement + disagreement) with a target rate of 85% reliability as the lowest acceptable level for each category [Miles & Huberman, 1994]. The software program ATLAS/ti was used to facilitate the inductive and deductive development and application of codes across data sources, as well as the creation of conceptual models.

## Separated-Reunited and Unaccompanied Minor Narratives

Below, we first describe the separation experiences of participants in the LISA study, followed by the separation experiences of unaccompanied minors in the ICAMA study. We will only highlight separation experiences of unaccompanied minors because they still remain separated from their families. We will conclude with revealing the reunification perspectives of the LISA study participants.

In the LISA study, the challenges of family separations emerged throughout our qualitative interviews whether from the perspectives of school personnel, immigrant youth, or their parents. Many people we met in school buildings noted the psychological consequences of separation experience as major hurdles for newcomer students to overcome in order to successfully adapt to the new school system. Immigrant youth and their parents testified painful experiences of separation and difficulties they went through upon reunification. By the end of 5 years of the longitudinal study, however, most families said that they found ways to come to terms with their feelings and learned how to live with each other again.

### The Perspective of School Personnel

During the course of our fieldwork, the issue of family separations and the subsequent reunifications was insightfully brought up as one of the challenges faced by immigrant students by a number of school personnel. Spontaneously, a high school counselor told us:

[In many cases] the family has been separated for many years . . . so when they are reunited sometimes it's a mess in the literal sense of the word. The mother doesn't know the child. . . Because she knows she's been working, sending money, caring for the child and everything – she's been doing her part. But now it is the child's turn, you know, to show understanding, to show appreciation. . . Sometimes the mother is in a new relationship. So that kid may be coming to a new family with other siblings and a step-parent.

The director of a high school international center talked about his concerns and summed up the challenge:

I feel like I need to give [students] a great deal of personal and emotional support in the transition they are making. . . .You know, the whole issue of family separations. There are a lot of emotional issues, which come into this. . . We have people here from China, from Brazil, from

Haiti, from Central America, and what is interesting is that they are all [talk about] the same issues. 'I don't know how to live with my [reunited] parent.'

As we talked further with this and several other school administrators and teachers as well as the youth and parents themselves, this issue of 'not knowing how to live with my parent' was substantially different from the classically expressed teenage angst. This was an expression of not knowing how to live with a parent who had essentially become a 'stranger' over the course of a protracted separation.

*The Perspectives of Stepwise Immigrant Families Regarding the Separation Phase*
During the course of the 5-year LISA study, we asked questions about a wide range of topics; none were more difficult to broach than family separations and reunifications. Many of our otherwise talkative participants became withdrawn and nearly monosyllabic when we posed questions about this topic. When we asked directly about this topic, most (76%) of our participants admitted that their family never discussed the time apart. Indeed, in many immigrant families, silence at home surrounded the years of separation. Below, we reveal what we learned about their experiences.

The Pain of Separation
The youth spoke emotionally about separating from their loved ones. In fact, the act of separation was often described as one of the hardest things about coming to the US. One 14-year-old Dominican girl said: 'The day I left my mother I felt like my heart was staying behind. Because she was the only person I trusted – she was my life. I felt as if a light had extinguished. I still have not been able to get used to living without her.' We found that leaving a parent behind in the country of origin was described as a particularly poignant loss for the youth.

Parents also spoke of the angst of separating from their children. In many cases, this happened when the children were infants and toddlers, a critical period for developing the attachment with the parent. The mother of a 13-year-old Central American boy shared: 'It was very hard above all to leave the children when they were so small. I would go into the bathroom of the gas station and milk my breasts that overflowed, crying for my babies. Every time I think of it, it makes me sad.' And while the parents told us that they hoped to reunite quickly with their children, the obstacles of money and documentation led to many protracted family separations. A Salvadoran mother of 3 told us:

I never thought it would be so long. But I had no choice. My husband had been killed and my children had no one else. I had to make the journey to El Norte [North America]. I left them with my mother hoping I could send for them in a few months but life here is so expensive. I sent money back every month to take care of them and saved every dollar I could and I spent nothing on myself. My life was better in El Salvador. Here I had no friends. I was always lonely. I missed my children desperately and my family. I worked all the time. But a safe crossing was so expensive for 3 children.

For parents, separation from their children was often compounded with a host of other challenges associated with their migration. These included barriers due to language and cultural differences, long working hours typically with low wages, displacement from familiar settings, and limited social support system. Lack of documentation and concerns about security added exponentially to the distress stemming from having the family torn apart. Separations were clearly exacerbated by lack of documentation, though many families were separated for other reasons as well. The reasons for prolonged separation varied from job conditions and prolonged working hours that did not allow the supervision parents wanted to provide or unsafe neighborhood conditions; in such situations grandparental care sometimes was viewed as a better option. Other times, biological parents were unduly optimistic in estimating how long it would take to earn the funds to establish a stable home in the new country and save enough for the tickets for the child or children; while concurrently sending back remittances to support the children and parents the cost of living in the homeland at the lowest end of the economic ladder proved discouraging. Sometimes, the problem had to do with unstable parental relationships; the stress of immigration could lead to the breakup of the parental dyad again slowing down bringing over the children. And, of course, more than one of these reasons were involved in prolonging the reunification.

Maintaining Contact from Afar
Parents, particularly mothers, maintained contact with their children (94%) through a series of strategies which included regular phone calls, the exchange of letters, critical remittances, the sending of photos and gifts, and occasionally return visits (when finances and documentation status allowed). Each one of these forms of contact played important roles in solidifying the memory of the absent parent over time.

The capacity to send remittances to support the children as well as other family members, though abstract in the child's mind, is the core motivation behind the majority of the parental absences. Few of the children (11%), however, seemed to have a clear sense of why their parents were absent. This 15-year-old Guatemalan girl was an exception: 'I remember that my grandparents would tell me that my parents had to go to work so they could send money.'

Children did recall the gifts that were sent, sometimes on special occasions in the form of money so they could buy what they liked and often in the form of lovingly selected items sent with visitors. A 12-year-old Mexican girl recounted: 'My parents would send dolls, necklaces, clothes, and perfume. Things they thought I would like. Once they sent press-on nails. They would send it with friends or uncles who were visiting our town.'

For some, the gifts may have served to salve the absence of the parent. A 12-year-old Mexican boy explained, 'They [grandparents] would say to me, "son, do you miss you mother?" I would say, "yes" and then go and play. With the video games I would forget everything.' At some level, this youth seemed to be caught up in the moment and may not have been focused on his mother's absence. He may simply have been captivated by videogames, as were many of his peers; the game might also have served as an escape to assuage sadness associated with the mother's absence.

This strategy of staying in touch by sending gifts may have been effective for some families; for many, the only feasible means of maintaining contact may have been through such material gifts. Nevertheless, a few children reported that it was not what they really wanted. For example, 14-year-old Chinese girl said, 'Even though he kept giving me new beautiful clothes – so what? I felt that he is my father, he should STAY with me, and see how I grow up', suggesting that no amount of material could replace the value of a parent's presence and active involvement in the child's daily life.

Pictures played a particularly important role in keeping the parent alive in the imaginary of the children in their absence. A 10-year-old Mexican girl confided: 'I would think about her. . . I used to cry in my room with my mother's picture.' While some children had memories of their parents, for others, their parents were little more than imaginary figures. For instance, a 16-year-old Guatemalan girl (whose mother left when she was 2 and was not to see her until 8 years later when her asylum papers where finally granted), told us: 'I would look at the pictures of my mother and I would think that I would like to meet her because I could not remember her. . . I would say, "what a pretty mom – I would like to meet her".' For a number of participants, the parents in the picture were parents in name only; children had little or no remembered first-hand experiences or memories of the parent serving in the role of day-to-day care.

Long-distance communication is difficult to maintain over the course of time, especially in long-term separations and for children whose parents left when they were very young; as the children grow up, the parent becomes something of an abstraction. As the mother of a 12-year-old Salvadorian boy explained:

> They lived with my mother in El Salvador. I left when they were babies. I spoke to the eldest once a month by phone. As the little one grew, I spoke to him, too. But since he didn't know me, our communication was quite short. I really had to pull the words out of him.

In listening to parents, it was evident that the absent child (or children) remained a daily sustaining and motivating presence in their lives. For children, however, the story was somewhat different. Especially for children involved in long-term separations, the story regarding parents was more one of out of sight, out of mind, perilously maintained by relatives and sporadic contact.

*Separation Perceptions of Unaccompanied Minors*
Adolescents experiencing unaccompanied minor migration faced the challenge of attending school full-time, while working to financially support themselves, and at times their family members in their countries of origin. This unique group of adolescents reported that while it was difficult to negotiate the demands of school, employment, and the responsibility of maintaining their families or themselves, they persevered by telling themselves that they could do it. These adolescents demonstrated their commitment to their family by making a sacrifice for their family. Nevertheless, their narratives highlighted the distance and strain that their parent-child relationships suffered because of the lack of sharing daily experience. They also emphasized how difficult life was without their parents. Still, unaccompanied minors' motivation resulted from understanding their own sacrifice, wanting to be successful in the US, and wanting to help and make their family proud.

The following themes stress the experiences of adolescents leading in immigration who have not yet reunited with their parents. These themes included adolescents' decision and reason to immigrate, what their separation was like, their adaptation to living without their parents – needing to work, and their relationships with their parents during separation.

Adolescents' Reasons to Immigrate
There were three main reasons for adolescents' immigration: sacrificing for their family (25%), seeking employment (25%), and either the adolescents' desire to learn English or go to US schools (25%). Twenty-five percent of adolescents listed two simultaneous reasons for immigrating to the US, for example, sacrificing for the family and seeking employment. Adolescents who immigrated to the US as a sacrifice for their family either came to the US to work and send money to their family or to study in the US and subsequently, through the adolescent's completion of a US education, the family could ultimately have a better life.

Manuel who was 16 years old when he immigrated to the US from Mexico told about the sacrifices he had been making for his family since he was 14 years old. He explained:

> My dad was in an accident. I had to start working at 14 years old to support my family. Well it wasn't as necessary for me to come here [referring to the US], but simply from over there I couldn't sustain my family. Well I don't know I also wanted to visit. And that was simply it. I now see that it is easier to sustain my family from here without my father having to work.

Lucia on the other hand, who immigrated to the US at age 14 from Nicaragua perceived her sacrifice in coming to US as one that prospectively would help her family in the future. She said:

> That one day I am able to succeed and could help them get ahead. That I have a better future than they were able to have by being here [referring to US]. To also help them [referring to her family] get ahead.

Separation Feelings and Perceptions
Like some 'stepwise' migrated youth in the LISA study, unaccompanied minors had an emotional response to being separated from their parents. They expressed feeling sadness and missing their parent and wished they were in the US with

them. For instance, Osmon, who emigrated from Honduras at age 17 stressed missing his mother and longed to return to Honduras to see her.

> I miss her a lot and my biggest longing is to return to Honduras to see her. And to see my other sister who is over there.

Their emotional responses were a normal reaction to being separated from their parents. When asked to reflect on what it would be like to reunite with their parents, some said they would be happy and expressed excitement at the prospect. Unaccompanied minors expressed a desire to return to their countries of origin. Adolescent's desire to return to their countries of origin was related to the challenges of living without parents and the issues that arose from the separation. For instance, for unaccompanied minors, being separated from their parent meant that not only they had to provide for themselves financially and for their families in their countries of origin, but also to make good decisions by themselves to promote their own success in the US. Ricardo who immigrated at the age of 16 from Mexico stressed the difficulties of living without his immediate family in the US and the responsibility of making the right choices for himself to guarantee his success. He explained:

> Because for me, that most difficult thing of being here would be that well that you are not with your family, that you have to try to live by yourself, that you have support, but it's not a very close support. Well . . . try to live like the best possible way you are able to live. And try to keep away from bad habits or those kinds of things – because in this country there is too much alcohol and drugs.

Another issue that arose for adolescents was the differences in relationships between their relatives in the US and those in their countries for origin. For instance, while the relatives they lived with attempted to guide them, adolescents shared that their relationships in the US were not the same in comparison with their relationships with their parents and other relatives in their countries of origin. They felt that their relationships were more distant, not as supportive in comparison to those they had in their country of origin, and felt like their relatives haven't done as much for them as their family in their countries of origin would have.

However, 5 of the 8 unaccompanied minors stressed that the relative they resided with took on a parental role for them. Unaccompanied minors resided with aunts, older siblings, and cousins in the US. For these youth, their surrogate caregiver was supportive of the adolescent, and attempted to provide guidance, advice, and monitor them in their parent's absence. They also shared that their parents expected that the relative they resided with take on this role during the parent's absence. For instance, Javier who immigrated from Mexico at the age of 16 stressed how his mom trusted his brother to take on such a role. He said: 'I am with my brother. My mom trusts that he will guide me because I am his younger brother.'

Additionally, Araceli who immigrated to the US from Mexico at age 17 stressed that her uncle assumed a parental role for her. She said:

> I don't live with my parents. I live with my aunt and uncle. So, my uncle is responsible for me. My uncle is like my father. My parents are in Mexico.

Surprisingly, when Ricardo is asked who he perceived was part of his family, he said that he considered his brothers, sister-in law, nephew and friends as part of his family. He perceived those he lived with in the US as family and qualified their relationship as beautiful because they mutually respected each other and tried to get along. He also described the relationship with his immediate family to be a relationship of the past. He said:

> Part of my family includes my brothers, sister in law, nephews, and friends. . . The relationship I have with my family members here [referring to US] is beautiful. We each respect each other. We try to get along. We have no problems. . . How was the relationship with [my family over there], it was beautiful. I was there with my mom, my siblings, we lived together very well.

### Adapting to Work and Working

Among the ICAMA study participants, unaccompanied minors made up the majority of those who discussed the need to adapt to their jobs and working. Some reported not having to work in their countries of origin and now in the US having the demand of work for supporting both themselves and (for some) remittances to their family. These adolescents reported working almost a full-time schedule between their after-school and weekend shifts. They unanimously shared how challenging it was to work, attend school, and complete homework. These adolescents were successful at managing school and work demands because they believed they could do it. Lucia described her adjustment to employment and having to provide for herself financially. She said:

> Here it is more difficult because in Nicaragua I didn't have to work, I did not have to worry about having money because my parents would give me some and they bought everything for me.

For these adolescents, the sacrifice of coming to the US without parents and desiring to make their parents proud motivated them in wanting to take full advantage of the opportunities available to them in the US. They also tended to look down on youth who had their parents in the US and when these youth weren't taking full advantage of their educational opportunities.

One adolescent who did not work full time reported that every day after school, she would join her aunt at work to help her clean offices. This was the way she demonstrated her gratefulness to her aunt for housing her and providing for her financially. Some adolescents stated that their main reason to immigrate was to work. After finding employment, they then found out that they could also study and enrolled in school. For instance, Ricardo stresses how he dedicated his efforts towards work, and then started school. He said: 'I dedicated myself to work and then I decided to come to school.' However, 2 out of the 8 unaccompanied adolescents stressed that the relative they lived with emphasized the need to attend school first before giving the adolescent permission to work.

## Change in Family Role and Family Obligation

Unaccompanied minors' role changed from child to breadwinner and primary provider for their family. In the majority of cases adolescents sent remittances to their family, and they voluntarily did it to help support their family. Javier shared how he would send money to his mother. He said:

> Here it's an advantage because I can help my mom because I work and every 15, 20 days I send her money.

Still in one unique case if the adolescent did not send money, his family would not have their basic needs met. While this adolescent stressed how challenging it was to work and go to school, he was committed and motivated to support his family. His narrative highlighted his obligation to his family. Manuel took on 'adult' like responsibilities when he was 14. He has been financially supporting his family since he was 14 years of age after his father had an accident, which affected his walking. He began working and left school to take on this responsibility while living in Mexico. He took this responsibility seriously, was proud of this duty and expressed his commitment to his family several times in the interview. For instance, he explained that he sacrificed his own needs for those of his family. He shared that he didn't give himself any luxuries such as a dressing well and owning a newer car because he did not want to sacrifice his family to do it. He said that his family came first and his desires were secondary. Interestingly, when Manuel was asked what his responsibilities were as a family member, he responded by saying:

> What are my responsibilities – better said what responsibilities don't I have. Right now I have to provide for them like my dad did in the past... right now I am responsible whether they eat or not.

Manuel further compared his family responsibilities with other youth's and his cousin. He fully understood what his family obligation was and to a degree seemed to express some remorse about having this responsibility at a young age. For instance, he stated:

> He does not have the same responsibility I have [referring to his cousin]. He has lived his life as he has wanted. He wastes his money. There are 3 boys, and his brother can help his dad and his dad is also able to work. They really do

not have as much responsibility as I do. So, if I don't help my family, who will?

He also stressed that other youth who have their parents in the US should appreciate what they have and the opportunity to just attend school. He said:

> They should appreciate the opportunity that is here, that many of them have their parents here, and now that they are here [referring to the US] they can accomplish so many things. And of course the first thing they do is just be on the street and nothing else. They don't work. The first thing they should do with this opportunity is study, they can do so much – but the first thing is to take advantage of the opportunity to study that their parent is giving them and do your very best.

Parent-Child Relationships

Even with the challenges unaccompanied minors encountered, some described good and unchanged relationships with their parents, while others perceived their relationships as distant/strained.

Thirty-seven percent of unaccompanied minors described their parent-child relationships as good or unchanged. Good parent-child relationships included such features as adolescents receiving advice from parents, identifying with and getting along with their parents, both parties supporting and confiding in each other, and an overall sense of unity. Adolescents with good parent-child relationship also stated that they had no problems with their parents, except for occasional disagreements. Respondents who described unchanged parent-child relationships said everything was 'the same' when asked whether things were different between them and their parents compared to how it was together in their countries of origin. The relationship being unchanged meant that adolescents still felt the same love and support from their parents, adolescents still loved their parents, parents still gave the adolescent advice, adolescents and their parents were still forthcoming with information even though they were separated, and they had no major problems. However, these adolescents reported some strain on a day-to-day basis because they are not living similar experiences. Estafania's description of her parent-child relationship was resonant of a good parent-child relationship:

> Well I would say that a good relationship, sometimes with my mom I find myself a lot. I really find myself with her, well with your parents. With my dad I also get along with him a lot, but sometimes well like he takes care of you a lot that sometimes he doesn't want a boy to talk to you and sometimes he would get mad. But it's a good relationship with my parents, we really haven't ever had any serious problems, we never have had them. Everything is good.

Osmon explained the ways that his relationship with his mother remained unchanged. He said:

> Nothing has changed. Well, my mom still provides the same support. And always gives me advice. There are no problems.

Nevertheless, Lucia described that her feelings and behaviors towards her parents remained unchanged, still she recognized the strain the relationship experienced because of the lack of daily sharing.

> The way I behave when I talk to them. The respect I have for them. The love I have for them. The way they give me advice [is the same]. … We don't share daily experiences, we talk once a week. And that's just a little bit of time. They are unable to see what I am doing [daily].

With distant/strained relationships, there was a decrease in adolescents' feelings of closeness with parents and strained relations in the forms of: (1) limits in the sharing of experiences and feelings with parents and (2) feelings that they and their parents didn't know one another as well as they would had they not been separated. The experience of living apart from their parents created for these adolescents a vagueness regarding parents' expectations. At times, unaccompanied minors reported that they no longer knew how to support their families. These adolescents were less forthcoming about information regarding their daily lives; they elected not to share their problems with their parents as they did not want to worry them. Manuel and Ricardo in their narratives stressed the strain and distance that unaccompanied minors experienced. Manuel said:

The relationship with my family is now just talking to them on the phone when they call. We talk about everything that is going on over there and what is going on with them. But, understandably if I have a problem here I don't tell them about it because they are only going to worry. It's not that I don't trust them, but they are going to worry, so I prefer not to say anything. . . [The relationship has changed] for the same reason that I am no longer over there, we don't see each other or talk to each other less. Regardless of how often we speak on the phone, it is not the same as being over there. We don't live together as we used to.

Ricardo reported that his existing relationships with his mother and siblings were close and good relationships. However, his descriptions of his relationships sounded distant and strained. He at times referred to the close relationship he 'had' with parents, especially his mom as one that was in the past. For instance, he said: 'how was the relationship with [them], it was beautiful. My mom is over there; with my mom and brothers we got along very well.' In another part of his story, he explained that he and his immediate family remained united, but acknowledged that there was distance and strain on the relationship because of the separation. Ironically, he explained that not being with his parents no longer affected him and if something happened to his mom it would not affect him as much because he is not as attached as he used to be. He said, 'Now I don't support them the same way because I am not there with them. So then I don't know how to help them. . . . Sometimes it does change a bit, I don't know like being away from them like it makes you feel that it doesn't affect you as much, I don't know. If at a certain point let's say my mom is no longer with me well I won't feel it as much because I am already a little used to not being as close to her.' This perhaps reflected the adaptation he had to make to survive in the US.

While unaccompanied minors faced the challenge of attending school full-time, working to financially support themselves, and at times their family members in their countries of origin, they remained motivated to support their families, succeed in the US, and make their family proud.

Nevertheless, their narratives also highlighted wanting to be with their parent to receive support and alleviate the daily demands of their lives. Some described the strain and distance their family relationships endured because of the separation.

### *The Perspectives of 'Stepwise' Immigrant Families Regarding the Reunification Phase*

One might expect that the reunification would be joyful. And indeed many children, especially those who had short-term separations or who had been separated only from one parent while living with the other, described the moment of reunification in positive terms (67%); notably the modal word choice was 'happy'. A 13-year-old Guatemalan girl said that on the day she got together with her mother: '[I was] so happy. It was my dream to be with her.' An 11-year-old Mexican boy said: 'I was very happy to be with my parents again.' Likewise, a Dominican 14-year-old girl described her family as they got together as: 'We were so happy. We cried, talked a lot and embraced.'

### Meeting a Stranger

Yet for many children who had endured protracted separations, the reunification was more complicated. In almost all cases, the children recalled that their parents, mothers in particular, received them in a highly emotional (sometimes tearful) but overwhelmingly welcoming (88%) manner. However, for them, as new arrivals, the parent was often described somewhat of a stranger (36%). As a Guatemalan 14-year-old girl recalled: 'My mother was crying. She hugged me. . . and I felt bad. Like neither my sister nor I knew her.' Thus, for immigrant children, the reunification meant entering a new life in a new land, often with a new set of adults whom they would call mother and father, or parents whom they have not seen for a long time.

Feelings of disorientation emerged frequently from the data. As a 13-year-old Haitian girl shared: 'I didn't know who I was going to live with or how my life was going to be. I knew of my father but I did not know him.' Even under optimal circumstances, migrating to a different country and adopting a new way of life is likely to be disorientating. Yet for many youth in our study, this adaptation process was further complicated by the uncertainty about whether they would feel comfortable in their own homes, get along with the people they would be living with, and what their routines in the home would be like. In essence, many of these youth were not only migrating to a new land but also to a new family and lifestyle.

At times, the children reported not recognizing the parent and described difficulties in forging a relationship with a near stranger. A 10-year-old Chinese girl recalls: 'The first time I saw my father, I thought he was my uncle. . . I was really afraid when I saw my father's face. He looked very strict. I was unhappy. My father was a stranger to me.' Similarly, a 13-year-old Guatemalan girl whose father left before her birth and whose mother left when she was a year old, not reuniting until 9 years later, told us:

> I felt something very strange and since I didn't know my mother I would see a lot of women [at the airport] and I didn't know who was my mom. And when she came to hug me, I said to her, 'Are you my mom?' I didn't hug her very strongly because I didn't know her or anything. I didn't have that much trust or didn't feel that comfortable with her.

Some parents perceived the gap in the trust. The mother of a 14-year-old Honduran boy told us: 'It was really hard at the beginning because we had been separated for 5 years. At the beginning, he barely trusted me, but now, little by little. . .' Thus, the effects of separation often lingered; the process of mending the relationship was a slow one. In most families, the healing process took 2 or 3 years. In a few of the most conflicted families, however, residual issue remained evident by the end of the 5 years of the longitudinal study.

In some cases, the predominant feeling expressed was of simple disorientation that needed time to heal. A 16-year-old Guatemalan girl, who had been separated since toddlerhood before reuniting with her mother 10 years later, told us: 'It felt weird calling her mom. I had to call her mom but it felt weird at first. Because I had called my grandparents mamí (mommy) and papí (daddy) for everything.'

For other adolescents, the extended absence led to a sustained rejection of the parent who they perceived to have had abandoned them (22%). In such cases, the damage of the long absence led to rifts that seemed challenging to traverse. A 14-year-old Chinese girl confided that after a 9-year absence: 'Suddenly I had another creature in my life called "father". . . I was too old by then and I could no longer accept him into my life.' For some youth, by the time parents reentered their life it was too late. These youth had grown accustomed to living without the missing parent; they were ready to assert greater independence and were unwilling to submit to the parents' authority after an extended absence.

Coming to Terms with New Family Members
Parents and adolescents both reported that reunifications could be complicated when the youth had to adapt to an entirely new family constellation. Discomfort with living with new step-parents (or partners) or a new sibling (or step-siblings) was frequently noted by both participants and their parents (26%). For example, this 12-year-old Mexican girl admitted that she had not wanted to migrate because: 'I did not know anybody and I was going to live with a man [a new step-father] I did not like.' And a 10-year-old Chinese girl confided that she had not 'expect[ed] to live with a stepmother'. Outright jealousy was also noted at times. The mother of a 13-year-old Nicaraguan boy disclosed:

> We are getting used to each other. We are both beginning a different life together. . . [T]he kids are jealous of each other and my husband is jealous of them. . . Jealousy exists between those who were born here and those who were not. My son says: 'You already spent a lot of time with her [his younger sister born in the US].'

This family, like many others in our study, had to negotiate multiple new relations. The mother needed to build her relationship not only with each of her children, but also maintain a healthy marriage. Furthermore, she was positioned to mediate her children's relationship with each other and the relationship between the children and her spouse. It was not unusual for the youth to particularly envy attention lavished on new siblings (or step-siblings), which they had not received in their parent(s)' absence. As a 14-year-old Chinese girl articulately stated: 'Now whenever I see how my father spends time playing with my younger sister, I always get mad that he never gave me fatherly love. Now I think he is trying to make [it] up to my younger sister.' Such envy often led to tension and conflict between family members.

Missing Caregivers in the Homeland
While reunification was often described as a happy event, it was often interlaced with contradictory emotions. The grief of loss is often re-experienced again upon reunification, when the children had to leave the caretaker (often a grandparent or aunts and uncles) who became the symbolic parent during the absence of the parent. A 16-year-old Guatemalan girl explained:

> I loved living with them [grandparents] because they were really sweet people. They were wonderful parents. For me they are not like grandparents, they are like my parents because they understand me, [and] they love me. . . I did not want to leave them. We were used to living with them.

Understandably, for many students in the study, the caregivers with whom they had daily physical contact had assumed an important role in their lives. An 11-year-old Salvadorian girl said: 'I left my aunt and uncle. I felt like they were my parents because they took care of me for 8 years.' This meant that for the migrating child, there was a bittersweet feeling upon reunification. A 16-year-old Guatemalan girl told us: 'I was sad because I had left my grandparents behind but happy to be together with my mother and all.' Similarly, an 11-year-old Central American boy told us: 'I was crying because I was leaving my grandfather. I had conflicting feelings. On the one hand I wanted to see my mother, but on the other I did not want to leave my grandfather.' Such separations and connections to caregivers were major disruptions to which students had to adapt (44%).

Most of the participants expressed sadness and resignation about the loss of their caretaker in the country of origin though on occasions, anger was the prevailing emotion (14%). A 14-year-old Chinese girl told us: 'I felt like they tried to rob me away from my grandmother. I felt like my father was the one who took me away from [her]. . . I always blame him for separating me and my grandmother.' A mother of a 9-year-old Mexican girl expressed the dilemma of missing parental figures succinctly: 'Before she came, she missed us. Now she misses her grandparents.' In these families, the grandparents also endured two major separations. The elderly had said good-byes to their own children when the family migration to the US began, and for a second time, they had to bid farewell to their grandchildren whom they had raised as their own children.

(Re)Establishing Authority
Parents often expressed tremendous guilt for being away from their children while recognizing that their sacrifice was necessary for the good of the family. At the same time, it often dawned on them that their children did not always understand this. Basic issues like parental authority and credibility was often undermined (38%) particularly with lengthy separations. An insightful mother of a 13-year-old Central American girl admitted:

> Our relationship has not been that good. We were apart for eleven years and communicated by letters. We are now having to deal with that separation. It's been difficult for her [my daughter] and for me. It's different for my son because I've been with him since he was born. If I scold him he understands where I'm coming from. He does not get angry or hurt because I discipline him but if I discipline her, she takes a completely different attitude than he. I think this is a normal way to feel based on the circumstance.

Children in such families likely perceived that their parents treated new siblings differently. This perception led to not only tensions between parent and child, but also to reported conflict between siblings and behavioral or emotional difficulties.

Was It Worth It?

We asked participants whether there was anything they would have liked to be done differently or if they thought it would have been better if their parents had stayed in their country of origin. The responses to these questions were revealing. Most indicated that they thought that their parents had made the right decision to migrate. As a 16-year-old Guatemalan girl acknowledged: 'If they had not left, we would be living like a lot of people over there who don't have any money.'

Nonetheless, nearly all the youth regretted the actual separation (82%): A 12-year-old Haitian boy wished, 'for the whole family to be together, [and that] we never separate again'. And a 16-year-old Guatemalan girl told us: 'I would have liked for all of us to have come together here with my grandparents and not suffered as we did when we were apart.'

Resilience in the Face of the Pain of Separations and Reunifications

Clearly, the migratory journey lead parents to make sacrifices to provide for their families; in the process, many were away for large portions of their children's formative years. For the immigrant parents, the children maintained a very real presence in their daily existences. Parents framed the daily rigors of their lives as a narrative of sacrifice for their children and dreamed of the longed-for-reunification as a way to sustain them through the painful separations. On the other hand, for the children who underwent lengthy separations, over time, the absent biological parent(s) began to fade to an abstraction. While parents were often appreciated and loved in their imagination, it was their daily caregivers who were their de facto parents. Children missed their parents, but most adapted to their caretaking situations especially if it happened early in their childhood, was over a sustained period of time, and was in a caring environment. In fact, the youth would later report missing their caregivers when they first arrived to their new land.

In the short-term, both parents and children reported that the reunification process was often difficult. This was especially true when the separation was a protracted one from both parents or from the mother. In these cases, the youth appeared to have substituted their attachments to their caregivers in the home country and thus sustained the double loss of homeland and parental figure in migrating. Over time, however, most of the participants appeared remarkably resilient. A 14-year-old Nicaraguan boy summed up what seemed to be the experience of many: 'The adaptation took a little time but we tried to get along and then little by little we became comfortable with one another.'

## Conclusions

In this chapter, we provided evidence on the impact of the separation and reunification experiences of 'stepwise' migrant families and the separation perspectives of unaccompanied minors using qualitative data from the LISA study [Suárez-Orozco et al., 2008] and the ICAMA study [Hernández, 2009]. The majority of immigrant children in the LISA sample had been separated from one or both parents. In the case of unaccompanied minors, they remained separated from both parents. With well over 20% of children in the US growing up in immigrant homes, the implications for numbers of youth affected by this phenomenon is striking [Hernández et al., 2007]. Of course, transnationally separated families are not unique to the US – post-industrial nations all over the world have experienced large scale migrations over the last decade [Bernhard et al., 2006; Gratton, 2007; Marks, 2005; UNDP, 2009]. Transitional family formations are increasingly becoming an issue of concern all over the world [Bohr et al., 2009; Bryceson &

Vuerola, 2002; Domingo, López-Falcon & Bayona Carrasco, 2010; Ryan, Sales, Tilki & Sciarra, 2009; UNDP, 2009]. Furthermore, broad socioeconomic transformations have stimulated large-scale internal migrations within nations. Countries like China, India, and Turkey among others have seen massive rural to urban migration bringing about similar patterns of displaced and separated families in disparate national settings [International Organization for Migration, 2008; Qin & Albin, 2010], which might present similar familial separations.

Certainly, the review of psychological consequences of separation and analyses of qualitative data clarified the poignancy of the process of separations from teachers', children's, and parents' points of view. Consistent with the findings of others [Charnley, 2000; Totternman, 1989], most children and youth whether stepwise migrants or unaccompanied minors reported missing their parents, although the losses resulting from the separations and the turmoil of reunification apparently did not lead to long-term psychological outcomes for stepwise migrant youth as measured by a standardized measure [Suárez-Orozco et al., 2011]. Nonetheless, family separations led to at least short-term angst for parents and children alike.

Our findings from the long-term patterns of psychological outcomes, however, [Suárez-Orozco et al., 2011] as well as the qualitative descriptions of the majority of the immigrant families about their relationships indicated that most newcomer stepwise immigrant youth appear to adjust to the loss and negative circumstances of separation resulting from migration over time. On the other hand, unaccompanied minors must continue to learn to adapt to the demands of living without the guidance of a parent, while navigating their employment, school work, distant parent relationships, and taking independent adult-like decisions. Still, unaccompanied minors seemed largely reconciled with their challenges by making meaning of their sacrifice by framing it as a desire to be successful in the US, as well as wanting to help and make their family proud.

While there were clearly adjustments and distress in the initial years of separations and reunification for stepwise immigrant families, psychological distress (as measured by a symptom checklist measure shortly after reunification and then again 5 years later) declined over the course of years. The qualitative retrospective data also had both youth and parents reporting that though the experience of separations had been painful, most had come to terms with the process. Both parents and youth described acute discomfort in the initial months and years following reunification, but in most cases remarkable strength, determination, resourcefulness, and resilience in adjusting to the clear challenges the separations and adjustments imposed by the reunification. Thus, immigrant youth in our study are remarkably resilient in coping with the painful experience of separation and the complications of adjusting to new family constellations. They ultimately learned to adapt to their new families and reformed relationships with their parents. This result is consistent with research that suggests many youth and families have a noteworthy capacity to overcome negative circumstances in their lives [Masten, 2001]. Our findings are also consistent with the argument that it is important to consider the perspective of time in examining adaptations to adversity [Luthar & Cicchetti, 2000].

Review of academic ramification of separations provided the opportunity to consider another important variable in youth's lives besides psychological symptoms. The existing literature and the analyses of our data [Suárez-Orozco et al., 2010a] suggest that having undergone a separation from the mother or father has a more deleterious influence on youth's academic adaptation in the host country. Thus, family separations appear to leave some students academically vulnerable. Given the prevalence of separations during migration, this is a deeply troublesome trend. While the psychological symptoms and problems in family relations may dissipate over time, undergoing significant length of family separations place some students at risk for academic difficulties down the road. For unaccompanied minors who elect to enroll in school after securing employment, they may have a difficult time managing their full time employment demands with school responsibilities, which often leads to temporarily dropping out of school. Separated youth may have fallen behind academically in anticipation of the migration or might not have gotten optimal academic supervision from grandparents or aunts prior to migration placing them academically behind as they enter the schools in their new homeland. They may also be suffering from lack of supervision or academic guidance at home. More research will be needed to unpack the reasons behind why separations leave adolescents particularly vulnerable academically.

Mitigating the separations and complicated reunifications, we identified protective factors such as attending better quality schools that are attentive to the needs of this population and having mentors who helped youth navigate their way through the educational system in the new land [Suárez-Orozco et al., 2008, 2011]. Through collaborative efforts, researchers and educators can identify protective factors and find ways to increase immigrant students' access to appropriate services and support which will help youth struggling from pains of family separations to successfully adjust in academic settings.

Lastly, as nations, we should reconsider the policies that impose family separations that sometimes last more than half a childhood. Currently, as President Obama has said, our immigration 'system is broken' [Obama, 2010]. There are no systematic queues for immigrant families to enter [Anderson, 2010], and there is no apparent political will in sight to legalize the 11 million undocumented immigrants currently living in the US. We have a massive deportation mechanism in place whereby 400 thousand people are being deported annually, many of whom have authorized children [Chaudry et al., 2010]; parents must make Solomonic decisions of whether to leave children behind daily. Thus, currently our national policies are set up to exacerbate immigrant family separations with worrisome developmental implications [Suárez-Orozco, Yoshikawa, Ternaishi & Suárez-Orozco, in press].

**Future Research**

Future studies should attempt to establish prevalence rates in other high intensity immigration settings across the globe (especially in large sending and receiving centers) and with other populations of immigrants. This line of inquiry would best be done involving researchers on 'both sides of the border'. More research will be required to further unpack the short- and long-term effects of separations. Multiple outcomes should be considered beyond depression and anxiety, including academic performance, trust, family relations and conflict, interpersonal relations, perceived competencies, family obligations, among others, as these outcomes may have been affected by disruptions in family relations. Studies should be conducted to identify particularly vulnerable stages of development for separations and subsequent reunifications.

In addition, future research will need to identify factors contributing to the emerging pattern of academic risk. It may be that children and youth, prior to migration, under the supervision of more permissive grandparents, or in anticipation of the migration to a new land, may disengage from school and fall behind academically, finding it hard to catch up. It may also be that the complicated reunification makes it hard for students to concentrate on their studies, and the parents no longer have authority over their children to demand that they engage in school. Most likely, it may be some combination of these factors. This problem of low achievement and academic disengagement among children and adolescents who have undergone prolonged separations needs to be better understood. The gendered pattern of underachievement among separated children and adolescents should also be examined.

Cross-cultural perspectives are critical in understanding these migration-related separations. Theories on parent-child relationship such as attachment theory would predict that family separations lead to negative psychological outcomes more at some times than others in a child's life. Such frames of reference are limited, given that they were developed by Western-trained psychologists with the constricted lens of understanding associated with that perspective. For example, multiple mother figures might be more prevalent in some of the sending communities. This leaves us with the question of whether such theories and principles might 'apply to *many, most, or all...* irrespective of their national or cultural contexts and irrespective of income, [and] education' [Arnett, 2008, p. 609].

To avoid imposition of ethnocentric outcomes, doing initial qualitative work with professionals in the country of origin, considering outcomes of concern noted within that context, would strengthen the constructs and instruments used. Culturally sensitive work should consider cultural norms of childcare and the meaning of collective values of family in different cultures that are closely related to family separation issues. We find that child fostering is a normative childcare practice in the Caribbean and African cultures. For Chinese immigrants, it is now a common practice to send infants back to China to be raised by grandparents until they are school age; they are then returned to birth parents to begin their education in Canada or the US [Bohr et al., 2009; Da, 2003; Gaytán et al., 2006]. For most other families, separation could be an intentional strategy to seek greater opportunities for children's futures as well as to secure and improve the family's collective position in the globalized economy of the 21st century, as we can see in cases of 'parachute children' [Orellana et al., 2001], or in the case of unaccompanied minors the need to seek employment to improve their life opportunities and those of their family.

As noted earlier, future research should take into consideration developmental patterns, as there are likely to be certain stages of development in which children may be more or less vulnerable for separation or reunification. Disentangling the child's age of separation and reunification, and their length of separation would help us better understand the impact of separation and reunifications on children's development. Additionally, further research should consider understanding the role that particular beliefs about life stage and adulthood have globally in shaping adolescents' decision to immigrate without their parents. Further qualitative research needs to be conducted to unpack the gendered processes behind the variations and nuanced sensitivities to separations from the mother or the father. Evidence-based intervention studies should be developed with the aim of attenuating the effects of separation for stepwise migration youth as well as developing strategies to help families manage the reunification process. For unaccompanied minors, these interventions should develop support systems to help adolescents cope with their various responsibilities, their ongoing separation from their parents and isolation.

On a cautionary note, there are significant ethical landmines in conducting this kind of research, as participants are often both emotionally vulnerable when they speak of their significant losses as well as legally vulnerable, since many have not achieved full documented status. Thus, researchers must proceed with extreme care as they move forward in conducting research in this important domain affecting many families in our evermore globalizing world.

In general, it appears that for many immigrant youth, irrespective of culture of origin, separations cause angst that may create at least a temporary challenge to family relations and development. Many children and families report that the process is difficult and leads to a sense of longing and missing one another. Children and youth articulate missing loved ones – parents (during the separation phase) and caregivers (during the reunification phase). Quite notably, however, transnational youths display extraordinary resilience in the face of the adversities of family separation. Moving forward, those serving immigrant communities should keep in mind the magnitude of the phenomenon of immigrant family separations. While recognizing the short-term challenges such experiences present for families and youth, service providers and researchers must check their cultural biases, assumptions, and expectations of what a 'typical' family looks like, refrain from pathologizing, and keep an open mind about the long-term implications of immigrant family separations.

## References

Abrego, L. (2009). Economic well-being in Salvadoran transnational families: How gender affects remittance practices. *Journal of Marriage and Family, 71*, 1070–1085.

Ambert, A.M., & Krull, C. (2006). *Changing families: Relationships in context.* Upper Saddle River: Pearson.

Anderson, S. (2010). *Family Immigration: The long wait to immigrate.* Arlington: National Foundation for American Policy. http://www.nfap.com/.

Arnett, J.J. (2008). The neglected 95%: Why American psychology needs to become less American. *American Psychologist, 63*, 602–614.

Arnold, E. (1991). Issues of reunification of migrant West Indian children in the United Kingdom. In J.L. Roopnarine & J. Brown (Eds.), *Caribbean families diversity among ethnic groups* (pp. 243–258). Greenwich, C.T.: Ablex Publishing.

Arnold, E. (2006). Separation and loss through immigration of African Caribbean women to the UK. *Attachment & Human Development, 8*, 159–174.

Artico, C.I. (2003). *Latino families broken by immigration: The adolescent's perceptions.* New York, N.Y.: LFB Scholarly Publishing.

Bernhard, J.K., Landolt, P., & Goldring, L. (2006). Transnational, multi-local motherhood: Experiences of separation and reunification among Latin American families in Canada. *CERIS, Policy Matters, 24*. Retrieved on July 15, 2009, from http://ceris.metropolis.net/PolicyMatter/2006/PolicyMatters24.pdf.

Bohr, Y., Whitfield, N.T., & Chan, J.L. (2009). *Transnational parenting: A new context for attachment and the need for better models: Socio-ecological and contextual paradigms.* Paper presented at the meeting of the Society for Research in Child Development, Denver.

Boti, M., & Bautista, F. (1999). *When strangers meet.* In National Film Board of Canada.

Bronfenbrenner, U., & Morris, P.A. (1998). The ecology of developmental processes. In R.M. Lerner (Ed.), *Handbook of child psychology* (5th ed., Vol. 1, pp. 993–1028). New York, N.Y.: Wiley.

Bryceson, D., & Vuorela U. (2002). The transnational families in the twenty-first century. In D. Bryceson & U. Vyorela (Eds.), *The transnational family: New European frontiers and global networks* (pp. 3–30). Oxford, UK: Berg.

Burke, A.W. (1980). Family stress and precipitation of psychiatric disorder: A comparative study among immigrant West Indian and native British patients in Birmingham. *International Journal of Social Psychiatry, 26*, 35–40.

Capps, R.M., Castañeda, R.M., Chaudry, A., & Santos, R. (2007). *The impact of immigration raids on America's children.* Washington D.C.: The Urban Institute.

Charnley, H. (2000). Children separated from their families in the Mozambique war. In C. Panter-Brick & M.T. Smith (Eds.), *Abandoned children* (pp. 111–130). Cambridge, UK: Cambridge University Press.

Chaudry, A., Pedroza, J., Castañeda, R.M., Santos, R., & Scott, M.M. (2010). *Facing our future: Children in the aftermath of immigration enforcement.* Washington, D.C.: Urban Institute.

Crawford-Brown, C., & Melrose, J. (2001). Parent-child relationships in Caribbean families. In N. Webb (Ed.), *Culturally diverse parent-child and family relationships: A guide for social workers and other practitioners* (pp. 107–130). West Port, CT: Ablex.

Da, W.W. (2003). Transnational grandparenting: Child care arrangements among migrants from the People's Republic of China to Australia. *Journal of International Migration and Integration, 4*, 79–103.

Domingo, A., López-Falcon, D., & Bayona Carrasco, J. (2010). Family reunion in the Barcelona Province, 2004–2008. *Migraciones, 27*, 11–47.

Dreby, J. (2007). Children and power in Mexican transnational families. *Journal of Marriage and Family, 69*, 1050–1064.

Dreby, J. (2009). Honor and virtue: Mexican parenting in the transnational context. *Gender and Society, 20*, 32–59.

Eccles, J.S., Midgley, C., Wigfield, A., Buchanan, C.M., Reuman, D., Franagan, C., & Iver, D.M. (1993). Development during adolescence: The impact of stage-environment fit on young adolescents' experiences in schools and in families. *American Psychologist, 48*, 90–101.

Falicov, C.J. (2007). Working with transnational immigrants: Expanding meanings of family, community, and culture. *Family Process, 46*, 157–171.

Foner, N. (2009). Introduction: Intergenerational relations in immigrant families. In N. Foner. (Ed.) *Across generations: Immigrant families in America* (pp. 1–20). New York, NY: New York University Press.

Forman, G. (1993). Women without their children: Immigrant women in the U.S. *Development, 4*, 51–55.

Gándara, P., & Contreras, F. (2010). *The Latino educational crisis: The consequences of failed policies.* Cambridge, MA: Harvard University Press.

Gaytán, F.X., Xue, Q., & Yoshikawa, H. (2006). *Transnational babies: Patterns and predictors of early childhood travel to immigrant mothers' native countries.* Paper presented at the annual National Head Start Research Conference, Washington.

Gindling, T., & Poggio, S. (2008). Family separation and reunification as a factor in the educational success of immigrant children. *UMBC Economics Department Working Papers.*

Gindling, T.H., & Poggio, S. (2009). Family separation and the educational success of immigrant children. *Policy Brief.* Baltimore, MD: University of Maryland.

Glasgow, G.F., & Gouse-Shees, J. (1995). Themes of rejection and abandonment in group work with Caribbean adolescents. *Social Work with Groups, 4,* 3–27.

Glick-Schiller, N., & Fouron, G. (1992). 'Everywhere we go, we are in danger': Ti Manno and the emergence of Haitian transnational identity. *American Ethnologist, 17,* 329–347.

Gratton, B. (2007). Ecuadorians in the United States and Spain: History, gender and niche formation. *Journal of Ethnic and Migration Studies, 33,* 581–599.

Hernández, M.G. (2009). *An exploratory narrative study of the migration patterns, parent-child relationships, and the adaptation of immigrant Central American and Mexican adolescents.* Unpublished doctoral dissertation, University of Wisconsin-Madison, Madison.

Hernández, D., Denton, N., & McCartney, S. (2007). *Family circumstances of children in immigrant families: Looking to the future of America.* New York, N.Y.: Guilford Press.

Hondagneu-Sotelo, P. (1992). Overcoming patriarchal constraints: The reconstruction of gender relations among Mexican immigrant women and men. *Gender and Society, 6,* 393–415.

Hondagneu-Sotelo, P. (Ed.) (2003). *Gender and U.S. immigration: Contemporary trends.* Berkeley, CA: University of California Press.

Hondagneu-Sotelo, P., & Avila, E. (1997). 'I'm here, but I'm there': The meanings of Latina transnational motherhood. *Gender & Society, 11,* 548–571.

International Organization for Migration (2008). *World migration.* Geneva, International Organization for Migration.

Lashley, M. (2000). The unrecognized social stressors of migration and reunification in Caribbean families. *Transcultural Psychiatry, 37,* 203–217.

Levitt, P. (2001). *The transnational villagers.* Berkeley, CA: University of California Press.

Lieblich, A., Tuval-Mashiach, R., & Zibler, T. (1998). *Narrative research: Reading, analysis and interpretation.* Thousand Oaks, CA: Sage Publications.

Luthar, S.S., & Cicchetti, D. (2000). The construct of resilience: Implications for interventions and social policy. *Development and Psychopathology, 12,* 857–885.

Martínez, I. (2009). What's age gotta do with it?: Understanding the age-identities and school-going practices of Mexican immigrant youth in New York City. *The High School Journal, 92,* 34–48.

Marks, G. (2005). Accounting for immigrant non-immigrant differences in reading and mathematics in twenty countries. *Ethnic and Racial Studies, 28,* 925–946.

Masten, A.S. (2001). Ordinary magic: Resilience processes in development. *American Psychologist, 56,* 227–238.

Mattis, J.S., Grayman, N.A., Cowle, S., Winston, C., Watson, C., & Jackson, D. (2008). Intersectional identities and the politics of altruistic care in a low-income, urban community. *Sex Roles, 59,* 418–428.

Menjívar, C., & Abrego, L. (2009). Parents and children across borders: Legal instability and intergenerational relations in Guatemalan and Salvadoran families. In Foner, N. (Ed.), *Across generations: Immigrant families in America.* (pp. 160–189). New York, NY: New York University Press.

Miles, M.B., & Huberman, M.A. (1994). *Qualitative data analysis: An expanded sourcebook* (2nd ed.). Thousand Oaks, CA: Sage Publications.

Morgan, C., Kirkbride, J., Leff, J., Craig, T., Hutchinson, G., & McKenzie, K., et al. (2007). Parental separation, loss and psychosis in different ethnic groups: A case-control study. *Psychological Medicine, 37,* 495–503.

Obama, B.H. (2010). President Obama on illegal immigrants and immigration reform. Washington: American University. http://latimesblogs.latimes.com/washington/2010/07/obama-text-illegal-immigrants-immigration-reform.html.

Ong, A. (1999). *Flexible citizenship: The cultural logics of transnationality.* Durham, NC: Duke University Press.

Orellana, M.F., Thorne, B., Chee, A.E., & Lam, W.S.E. (2001). Transnational childhoods: The participation of children in processes of family migration. *Social Problems, 48,* 572–591.

Orfield, G., & Lee, C. (2006). *Racial transformation and the changing nature of segregation.* Cambridge, MA: The Civil Rights Project at Harvard University.

Partida, J. (1996). The effects of immigration on children in the Mexican-American community. *Child and Adolescent Social Work Journal, 13,* 241–254.

Qin, J., & Albin, B. (2010). The mental health of children left behind in rural China by migrating parents: A literature review. *Journal of Public Mental Health, 9,* 4–16.

Rong, X.L., & Preissle, J. (1998). *Educating immigrant students: What we need to know to meet the challenges.* Thousand Oaks, CA: Corwin Press.

Rousseau, C.I., Hassan, G., Measham, T., Moreau, N., Lashley, M., Castro, T., & McKenzie, G. (2009). From the family universe to the outside world: Family relations, school attitude, and perception of racism in Caribbean and Filipino adolescents. *Health & Place, 15,* 751–760.

Ruhm, C.J. (2004). Parental employment and child cognitive development. *Journal of Human Resources, 39,* 155–192.

Rutter, M. (1971). Parent-child separation: Psychological effects on the children. *Child Psychology and Psychiatry, 12,* 233–260.

Ryan, L., Sales, R., Tilki, M., & Siara, B. (2009). Family strategies and transnational migration: Recent Polish migrants in London. *Journal of Ethnic and Migration Studies, 35,* 61–77.

Scalabrini Migration Center (2003). *Heart apart: Migration in the eyes of Filipino children.* Quezon City: Scalabrini Migration Center.

Sciarra, D.T. (1999). Intrafamilial separations in the immigrant family: Implications for cross-cultural counseling. *Journal of Multicultural Counseling and Development, 27,* 30–41.

Sewell-Coker, B., Hamilton-Collins, J., & Fein, E. (1985). West Indian immigrants. *Social Casework, 60,* 563–568.

Small, S., & Covalt, B. (2006). The role of the family in promoting adolescent health and development: Critical questions and new understandings. In F.A. Villarruel & T. Luster (Eds.), *The crisis in youth mental health: Disorders in adolescence* (pp. 1–25). Westport, C.T.: Praeger Publishers.

Smith, R. (2006). *Mexican in New York: Transnational lives of new immigrants.* Berkeley, CA: University of California Press.

Smith, A., Lalonde, R.N., & Johnson, S. (2004). Serial migration and its implications for the parent-child relationship: A retrospective analysis of the experiences of the children of Caribbean immigrants. *Cultural Diversity and Ethnic Minority Psychology, 10,* 107–122.

Strauss, A., & Corbin, J. (1990) *Basics of qualitative research: Grounded theory procedures and techniques.* Thousand Oaks, CA: Sage Publications.

Suárez-Orozco, C., Bang, H.J., & Kim, H.Y. (2011). I felt like my heart was staying behind: Psychological implications of family separations & reunifications for immigrant youth. *Journal of Adolescent Research, 26,* 222–257.

Suárez-Orozco, C., Bang, H., & Onaga, M. (2010a). Contributions to variations in academic trajectories amongst recent immigrant youth. *International Journal of Behavioral Development, 34,* 500–510.

Suárez-Orozco, C., Gáytan, F.X., Bang, H.J., Pakes, J., O'Connor, E., & Rhodes, J. (2010b). Academic trajectories of newcomer immigrant youth. *Developmental Psychology, 46,* 602–618.

Suárez-Orozco, C., Suárez-Orozco, M.M., & Todorova, I. (2008). *Learning a new land: Immigrant students in American society.* Cambridge, MA: Harvard University Press.

Suárez-Orozco, C., Todorova, I., & Louie, J. (2002). 'Making up for lost time': The experience of separation and reunification among immigrant families. *Family Process, 41,* 625–643.

Suárez-Orozco, C., Yoshikawa, H., Teranishi, R., & Suárez-Orozco, M.M. (in press). Growing up in the shadows: The developmental implications of unauthorized status. *Harvard Education Review.*

Suro, R. (2003) *Remittance senders and receivers: Tracking the transnational channels.* Washington, D.C.: Multilateral Investment Fund and the Pew Hispanic Center.

Tyyska, V. (2007). Immigrant families in sociology. In J.E. Lansford, K.D. Deater-Deckard & M.H. Bornstein (Eds.), *Immigrant families in contemporary society.* New York, NY: Guilford Press.

United Nations Development Programme (2009). Human development report 2009 — Overcoming barriers: Human mobility and development. New York: United Nations Development Programme.

US Census Bureau (2000). Census 2000 summary. Retrieved from June 1, 2009 from http://factfinder.census.gov /servlet/ QTTable?_bm=y&-geo_id=01000US&-qr_name=DEC_2000_SF3_U_ QTP22&-ds_name=DEC_2000_SF3_U.

US Department of Health and Human Services, Administration for Children and Families, Office of Refugee Resettlement (2009). DHS UAC Apprehensions placed in ORR/DUCS care, by 2009 by state. http://www.acf.hhs.gov/programs/orr/ programs/unaccompanied_alien_children.htm.

Waters, J.L. (2002). Flexible families?: 'Astronaut households' and the experience of lone mothers in Vancouver, British Columbia. *Social & Cultural Geography, 3,* 117–134.

Wexler Love, E. (2010). *Aspirations, involvement, and survival: Immigrant Latino youth navigating school and community.* Unpublished doctoral dissertation. University of Colorado at Boulder.

Wilkes, J.R. (1992). Children in limbo: Working for the best outcome when children are taken into care. *Canada's Mental Health, 40,* 2–5.

Wong, B.P. (2006). Immigration, globalization and the Chinese American Family. In J.E. Lansford, K.D. Deater-Deckard & M.H. Bornstein (Eds.), *Immigrant families in contemporary society.* New York, NY: Guilford Press.

Wright, C.L. (2010). Parental absence and academic achievement in immigrant students. *FIU Electronic Theses and Dissertations. Paper 322.* http://digitalcommons. fiu.edu /etd/322

Zhou, M. (2009). Conflict, coping, and reconciliation: Intergenerational relations in Chinese immigrant families. In N. Foner (Ed.), *Across generations: Immigrant families in America.* (pp. 21–46). New York, NY: New York University Press.

Zhou, M. (1998). 'Parachute kids' in Southern California: The educational experience of Chinese children in transnational families. *Educational Policy, 12,* 682–704.

Prof. Carola Suarez-Orozco
NYU Steinhardt School of Culture, Education, and Human Development
726 Broadway, 5th Floor
New York, NY 10003 (USA)
E-Mail cso2@nyu.edu

# Author Index

Abubakar, A. 49
Arasa, J. 49

Chasiotis, A. 35

Dimitrova, R. 35

Gagné, M.H. 17
Garcia Coll, C. VII

Hernández, M.G. 122
Horenczyk, G. 64

Law, D.M. 17
Li, J. 1

Mazrui, L. 49
Murugami, M. 49

Oh, S.S. 77

Sam, D.L. 64
Shapka, J.D. 17
Suárez-Orozco, C. 122

van de Vijver, F.J.R. 49
van Geel, M. 99
Vedder, P. 99

Yamamoto, Y. 1
Yoshikawa, H. 77

# Subject Index

Acculturation
    adaptation definition 68
    cluster analysis of immigrant youth 65
    English proficiency and acculturation impact in Asian immigrants 7, 8
    ethnic identity relationship 50, 51, 53, 54, 58–60
Albanian immigrants, *see* Italy immigration
Arab immigrants, *see* Kenya immigration
Asian immigrant children
    cultural norms and school experiences 2, 3
    demographics 2
    Kenya, *see* Kenya immigration
    quietness
        consequences
            accultural stress 12
            peer acceptance 11, 12
            teacher interaction 10, 11
        overview 3, 4
        preschool Chinese children study
            design 5–7
            developmental indications 12, 13
            English proficiency and acculturation impact 7, 8
            limitations of study 13, 14
            subgroup analysis 8–10
            teacher perspective 7, 8
        Western self-expression adjustment 4, 5

Canada immigration
    adolescents
        British Columbia study
            covariates 27
            data analysis 23, 24
            limitations of study 30
            participant characteristics 22, 23
            peer similarity perception at school 23
            research questions 22, 24
            school social context impact 29, 30
            sense of belonging at school 23–29
            social support perception at school 23, 26, 27
        prospects for study 31
        school social context
            language 20, 21
            racial/ethnic perceptions 20
        sense of belonging 19, 20
        social support
            adults and teachers 21
            peers 21
    immigration paradox 18, 19
    rates 17
Childhood Social Adjustment Capacity Indicators Questionnaire-Self Report 40
Children's Depression Inventory 40
Chinese immigrants, *see* Asian immigrant children

Discrimination
    coping
        anger suppression and expression 107, 108
        discrimination as stressor 103, 104
        ethnic identity and self-esteem 104–106
        social support 106, 107
    education inequality 101–104
    health impact 100, 101
    multicultural education and discrimination
        approaches for study 108, 109
        ethnic identity and support 111, 112
        relationship improvement 109–111
        study on effects of school multiculturalism
            goals 113, 114
            implications 116, 117
            instruments 111

limitations of study  116
participant features  111
relation between perceived school multicultural atmosphere, discrimination, and well-being  114–116
school evaluation  114

English proficiency, acculturation impact  7, 8
Ethnic identity
    acculturation relationship  50, 51, 53, 54, 58–60
    discrimination coping  104–106, 111, 112
    Kenya immigrants  53, 54, 56, 57, 59, 60
    Multi-Group Ethnic Identity Measure  55, 61, 70

Family separation
    features in immigrant families  122, 123, 124
    Immigrant Central American and Mexican Adolescent study
        data sources
            coding of data  131, 132
            final interview  131
            follow-up interview  131
            initial interview  131
        design  130
        participants  130
    Longitudinal Immigrant Student Adaptation study
        data sources
            coding of data  131, 132
            follow-up interviews  130
            open-ended questions  129, 130
            school personnel interviews  130
        design  129
        immigrant family perspective regarding separation phase
            maintaining contact from afar  134
            overview  133
            pain of separation  133
        participants  128, 129
        resilience in separation and reunification  142
        reunification phase
            authority establishment  141
            meeting a stranger  139, 140
            missing caregivers in homeland  141
            new family member coping  140, 141
            regrets  142
        school personnel perspectives  132, 133
        unaccompanied adolescent perspective
            family role and obligation changes  137, 138
            overview  135
            parent-child relationships  138, 139
            reasons for immigration  135, 136
            work adaptation by adolescents  136, 137
    prevalence  124, 125
    prospects for study  144, 146
    youth experience in separations and reunifications
        academic adaptation implications  127, 128
        changes in family relations  125, 126
        psychological consequences  127

General Health Questionnaire-12  55, 56

Immigrant Central American and Mexican Adolescent study
    data sources
        coding of data  131, 132
        final interview  131
        follow-up interview  131
        initial interview  131
    design  130
    immigrant family perspective regarding separation phase
        maintaining contact from afar  134
        overview  133
        pain of separation  133
    participants  130
    resilience in separation and reunification  142
    reunification phase
        authority establishment  141
        meeting a stranger  139, 140
        missing caregivers in homeland  141
        new family member coping  140, 141
        regrets  142
    unaccompanied adolescent perspective
        family role and obligation changes  137, 138
        overview  135
        parent-child relationships  138, 139
        reasons for immigration  135, 136
        work adaptation by adolescents  136, 137
Immigration paradox  18, 19, 36
International Comparative Study of Ethnocultural Youth
    aims  65
    cluster analysis of acculturation by immigrant youth  65
    immigrant youth identity and adaptation based on society type

comparison of society types 74
Multi-Group Ethnic Identity Measure 70
participant features 69
psychological adaptation 70–72
sociocultural adaptation 70, 72
Italy immigration
   Albanian, Serbian, and Slovene immigration study
      children's adjustment outcomes
         ethnic differences 41, 42, 45, 46
         gender differences 41–43, 45
         social versus psychological adjustment outcomes 43, 44
      design 40
      instruments
         Children's Depression Inventory 40
         Childhood Social Adjustment Capacity Indicators Questionnaire-Self Report 40
      limitations of study 45, 46
      participant features 38–40
      research question 38
      self-ratings versus teacher reports 44, 45
   demographics 37
   overview 35–37

Kenya immigration
   acceptance of immigration 51
   adolescent immigrant study
      acculturation orientation 57–60
      ethnic identity and well-being 56, 57, 59, 60
      measures
         ethnic label 54, 55
         General Health Questionnaire-12 55, 56
         life satisfaction 55
      participant features 54
      research questions 54
   Arabs 52
   Asians 52, 53
   ethnic identity and accultural orientations 53, 54
   prospects for study 61
   Somalians 53

Longitudinal Immigrant Student Adaptation study
   data sources
      coding of data 131, 132
      follow-up interviews 130
      open-ended questions 129, 130
      school personnel interviews 130

   design 128, 129
   immigrant family perspective regarding separation phase
      maintaining contact from afar 134
      overview 133
      pain of separation 133
   participants 128, 129
   resilience in separation and reunification 142
   reunification phase
      authority establishment 141
      meeting a stranger 139, 140
      missing caregivers in homeland 141
      new family member coping 140, 141
      regrets 142
   school personnel perspectives 132, 133
   unaccompanied adolescent perspective
      family role and obligation changes 137, 138
      overview 135
      parent-child relationships 138, 139
      reasons for immigration 135, 136
      work adaptation by adolescents 136, 137

Migration morbidity hypothesis 35, 36
Multi-Group Ethnic Identity Measure 55, 61, 70

Quietness, Asian immigrant children
   consequences
      accultural stress 12
      peer acceptance 11, 12
      teacher interaction 10, 11
   overview 3, 4
   preschool Chinese children study
      design 5–7
      developmental indications 12, 13
      English proficiency and acculturation impact 7, 8
      limitations of study 13, 14
      subgroup analysis 8–10
      teacher perspective 7, 8
   Western self-expression adjustment 4, 5

Religion, *see* Spirituality
Reunification, *see* Family separation

Selective-migration hypothesis 35
Serbian immigrants, *see* Italy immigration
Settler societies
   cultural diversity 67

immigrant youth identity and adaptation based on society type
    comparison of society types 74
    Multi-Group Ethnic Identity Measure 70
    participant features 69
    psychological adaptation 70–72
    sociocultural adaptation 70, 72
immigration acceptance 66, 67
overview 66

Slovene immigrants, *see* Italy immigration
Societies of settlement, *see* Settler societies
Somalian immigrants, *see* Kenya immigration
Spirituality
    demographic and policy contexts of immigration, religion, and spirituality 78, 79, 94, 95
    spiritual capital
        characteristics 80, 81
        community perspectives
            faith-based organizations 92–94
            immigrant worship community characteristics 90, 91
            private religious schools 91, 92
        definition 79, 80
    developmental significance and stages 78, 83–86
    ethnic social networks, fictive kinship, and peer influences 89, 90
    family settings
        religious beliefs 86, 87
        spiritual and religious socialization 87–89
    predictors
        family history 81, 82
        individual disposition 81
        macrosystem forces 82, 83
    prospects for study 94, 95

Teachers
    family separation perspectives 132, 133
    Italy immigration study, self-ratings versus teacher reports 44, 45
    quietness of immigrant student
        effects on interaction 10, 11
        preschool Chinese children study 7, 8
    social support effects on Canada immigrants 21